HEMATOLOGY

Susan M. Cotter, DVM
Diplomate ACVIM (Internal Medicine and Oncology)

Distinguished University Professor
School of Veterinary Medicine
Tufts University
North Grafton, MA

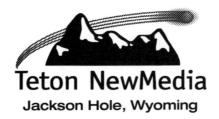

Teton NewMedia
Jackson Hole, Wyoming

Executive Editor: Carroll C. Cann
Development Editor: Susan L. Hunsberger
Editor: Cynthia J. Roantree
Typeset by Achorn Graphics, Worcester, MA
Printed by McNaughton & Gunn, Saline, MI
Illustrations by Anne Rains
Design and cover by Anita Sykes

Teton NewMedia
P.O. Box 4833
125 South King Street
Jackson, WY 83001
1-888-770-3165
http://www.tetonnm.com

The author and publisher have made every effort to provide an accurate reference text. However, they shall not be held responsible for problems arising from errors or omissions, or from
misunderstandings on the part of the reader.

Library of Congress Cataloging-in-Publication Data
Cotter, Susan M., 1943-
    Hematology / Susan M. Cotter.
      p.; cm.—(Quick look series in veterinary medicine)
    Includes bibliographical references and index.
    ISBN 1-893441-36-9 (alk. paper)
    1. Veterinary hematology. I. Title. II. Series.
    [DNLM: 1. Hematologic Diseases—veterinary. 2. Veterinary Medicine. SF 769.5
C847h 2001]
SF769.5 .C68 2001
636.089′615—dc21

                                                                    00-066646

PRINTED IN THE UNITED STATES OF AMERICA

ISBN 1-893441-369

Print number 5 4 3 2 1

Table of Contents

Dedication

To my husband, Richard H. Seder MD, MPH, for his love, support, friendship and expert professional advice.

To my colleagues and students who keep my profession exciting, and who challenge me to keep learning.

Preface

I have been active as a small animal medicine clinician, clinical researcher, and teacher for 34 years. After a few years in general medicine, I began to focus my interests in hematology and oncology. I joined the faculty at Tufts just after the veterinary school opened so that I could spend more time teaching residents and veterinary students. I took on the task of designing and teaching the Pathophysiology of the Hematopoietic System as a second year course, and Clinical Hematology in the third year Small Animal Medicine course. This provided a wonderful opportunity for me to review, organize and attempt to explain these concepts to students. I wrote my course syllabus and updated it annually since there was no basic student-oriented textbook for veterinary hematopoietic pathophysiology. The syllabus served as a starting point for this book.

When I was approached to write for the *Quick Look Series,* I was glad to take on the project. Now I had an opportunity to use my approach to this topic and take advantage of the artistic talent of Anne Rains to clarify what I was describing. This book contains only a small fraction of the rapidly expanding knowledge base in Veterinary Hematology. The reader is referred to some of the references listed at the end to learn more. However, if the reader becomes familiar with the majority of the information in this book, he or she will be able to understand the mechanism for the most common hematologic abnormalities that occur. This will provide the basis for an approach to veterinary patients with these diseases.

Veterinarians deal with many species, among which there are certain similarities and differences. At times, students can become overwhelmed trying to remember species-specific details. As much as possible in this book, I have emphasized those aspects that are common to most domestic animals and to man. Where important differences exist, I have mentioned those. Information presented without mention of species can be assumed to be essentially true for all.

As a clinician I have tried whenever possible to explain the clinical relevance of each topic. Some reference is made of treatment, although that is covered in more detail in medicine texts.

Overall I think of this book as a beginning. I hope it will stimulate students, interns, residents, practicing veterinarians, and researchers to want to learn more. Please let me know if you note any major omissions or errors.

Susan M. Cotter

Acknowledgments

I would like to thank Jim and Matt Harris for the original idea for the *Quick Look Series,* Dr Jim Ross at Tufts for his enthusiasm and encouragement in this project, and especially Carrol Cann and Susan Hunsberger at Teton NewMedia for their expertise in putting it all together.

HEMATOLOGY

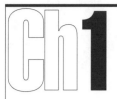

Components of Blood

A Types and Function of Plasma Proteins

Protein	Function
Albumin	Osmotic function; major carrier protein

Globulins
 	
α_1–Antitrypsin
 	
α_2–Macroglobulin
α_2–Antiplasmin
Antithrombin
 	
Haptoglobin
Lipoproteins
Transferrin
Fibrinogen
Plasminogen
Clotting factors
Immunoglobulins
	Inhibits trypsin and other proteases such as
	   kallikrein, plasmin, thrombin
	Immunoregulatory, protease inhibitor
	Inhibits plasmin
	Activated by heparin to inactivate thrombin and
	   other clotting factors
	Binds and transports free hemoglobin
	Transports lipids
	Binds and transports iron
	Clotting factor; acute-phase reactant
	Precursor to fibrinolytic protease
	All factors and other inhibitors
	Includes β– and γ–globulins produced by
	   plasma cells

B Preparation of Blood Smear for Differential White Blood Cell Count

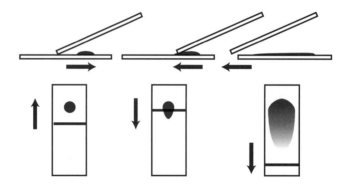

C Microscopic Appearance of Stained Blood Smear

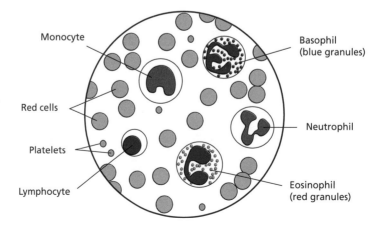

Blood makes up 5%–7% of the body weight, and about 60% of the blood volume is plasma and 40% cellular elements. Blood serves as a transport system for cells, proteins, and other substances dissolved in plasma, and maintains the hydration and oxygenation of all tissues of the body. The blood also transports glucose and fatty acids for nutrition, enzymes, hormones, and ions such as sodium, hydrogen, potassium, calcium, magnesium, chloride, and bicarbonate, as well as delivers drugs and removes waste products.

Plasma Proteins

Most proteins are synthesized in the liver. A partial list of major plasma proteins is provided in **Part A**. Three classes of proteins are present in the plasma: carrier proteins, immunoproteins, and coagulation proteins. Albumin, a carrier protein, makes up about two-thirds of the mass of plasma proteins and has a half-life in the dog of approximately 8–9 days. Albumin, because of its small molecular size (about 66,000 d), and sodium are the major sources of osmotic pressure, needed to maintain plasma volume and regulate diffusion of water from the vascular space into the tissues.

Albumin is relatively conserved in states of malnutrition at the expense of other body proteins such as those in muscle. Only in the setting of severe malnutrition does serum albumin concentration begin to decrease. No known disease causes an increase in albumin concentration, so animals with a high albumin concentration are likely to be dehydrated. The loss of fluid causes only a relative increase in albumin.

Albumin may be lost through the kidneys or intestines in some disease states. Glomerulonephritis and renal amyloidosis cause leakage of albumin through the glomerulus into the urine. Albumin can also be lost into the intestines in some inflammatory diseases or lymphangiectasia. In some maldigestion and malabsorption intestinal diseases, amino acids are not absorbed and proteins are not made. Usually diarrhea is a prominent sign, but it may be absent. Bleeding into the gastrointestinal tract will result in the loss of both red blood cells and protein, so hypoproteinemia and anemia occur. A difference between renal and intestinal protein loss is that glomerular lesions preferentially leak albumin, whereas in intestinal diseases, all protein levels may be decreased.

Because albumin is synthesized entirely in the liver, it can be used as an indicator of hepatic function. Hypoalbuminemia from liver disease almost always is accompanied by other signs specific to the liver, and a decrease of albumin usually is seen only in severe and chronic hepatic dysfunction. Regardless of the cause of hypoalbuminemia, the clinical signs are associated with loss of oncotic pressure in the plasma, and leakage of fluid into tissues and body cavities. Patients may have peripheral or pulmonary edema, ascites, or pleural effusion.

The other major components of plasma proteins are the globulins, which function as carrier proteins, immunoglobulins, inhibitors, and coagulation factors. Examples of carrier proteins are lipoproteins, which transport cholesterol; transferrin, which carries iron to developing red blood cells in the marrow; haptoglobin, which binds free hemoglobin released from damaged red blood cells; and various antitrypsins, antiproteases, and macroglobulins, which bind and remove proteolytic enzymes and moderate the effects of inflammation in tissues. Immunoglobulins and complement play an important role in the humoral immune response.

The last major group of proteins is involved in coagulation and anticoagulation. When blood is withdrawn from the body, it will immediately clot unless an anticoagulant is added. The liquid remaining after blood clots is called *serum*. Serum differs from plasma in that certain coagulation factors are removed. Once coagulation is complete, other circulating anticoagulants begin to limit further coagulation by inactivating factors, while other substances such as plasmin begin to break down fibrin.

Blood Cells

Red blood cells (erythrocytes) are the most numerous, comprising $5–6 \times 10^6$ cells/μL in humans and most mammals. They make up approximately 45% of the blood volume. The volume of red blood cells can be calculated by an automated cell counter and is referred to as the *hematocrit* (Hct). Mature mammalian red cells have lost their nucleus while those of other vertebrates are nucleated. Red cells in common domestic animals have the shape of a biconcave disk although there is some variation in shape and size. (*See* chapter 58 for reference ranges for various species.) The function of red cells is to pick up oxygen in the lungs and deliver it to the tissues. Mature mammalian red cells provide the maximum surface area per volume, for ease of oxygen transfer to and from the cell. Red cells function entirely within the vascular space.

The function of white blood cells (leukocytes) is to defend against infection or other "foreign" invaders such as tumor cells. The white cells are divided into phagocytes, which can engulf foreign matter, and lymphocytes, which are part of the immune system. White cells travel in the blood to the tissues where they perform their various functions. Most types of white cells, with the exception of lymphocytes and possibly monocytes, cannot return to the circulation after they leave. In the circulation, a normal white blood cell count is roughly $5–15 \times 10^3$ cells/μL. Changes in the numbers of each type of white cell have clinical significance.

Platelets are enucleated cytoplasmic fragments of megakaryocytes and are the first line of defense against blood loss. Platelets adhere to damaged areas of the endothelium to form a plug, on which fibrin forms. A normal platelet count for most animals is $2–4 \times 10^5$ cells/μL.

The cellular elements of the blood are easily examined on a blood smear. A drop of blood is placed on a slide, smeared with a second slide (**Part B**) and stained (**Part C**).

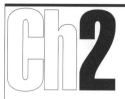

Hematopoiesis

A   Normal Hematopoiesis

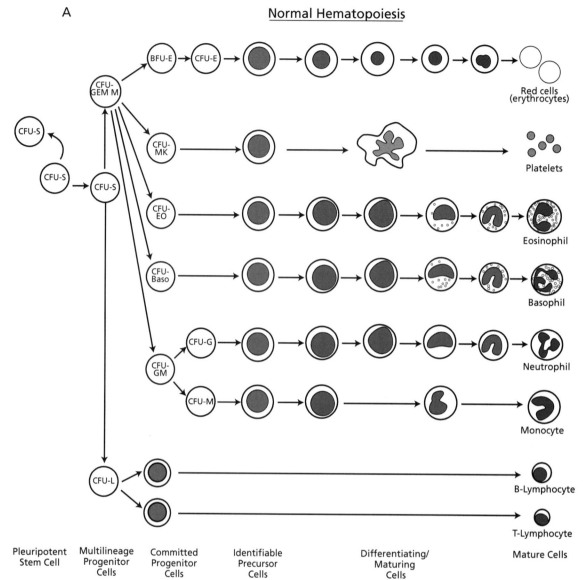

| Pleuripotent Stem Cell | Multilineage Progenitor Cells | Committed Progenitor Cells | Identifiable Precursor Cells | Differentiating/ Maturing Cells | Mature Cells |

B   Relative Numbers of Marrow Hematopoietic Cells

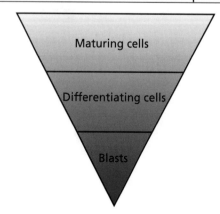

Blood cells must be replaced constantly. Neutrophils travel to tissues within hours of entering the circulation and never return. Platelets survive approximately 1 week but are consumed as they plug up leaks in blood vessels. Red cells survive in the circulation for 3–4 months, depending on the species.

Hematopoiesis is the process during which mature red and white blood cells and platelets are produced in the extravascular compartment within the marrow cavity. To maintain appropriate numbers, complex cellular and humoral interactions regulate the proliferation, differentiation, and maturation of each cell type. Bone marrow stem cells give rise to a pool of progenitor cells, which are committed to the differentiation of many cell types; the specific cell type developed depends on which growth factors and colony-stimulating factors (CSFs) are present (**Part A**).

The formation of new blood cells also requires a favorable marrow microenvironment, and adequate nutrition.

Development of the Bone Marrow

The yolk sac is the initial site of hematopoiesis. As the fetus matures, first the liver, then the spleen, and finally the marrow begin to produce blood cells. At the time of birth, the medullary cavity of most bones contains active marrow. As an animal matures to adulthood, active marrow becomes fairly localized to the bones of the axial skeleton, e.g., the vertebrae, sternum, ilium, ribs, and the proximal and distal ends of long bones. The marrow can increase its production of any type of blood cell whenever the need arises. Effective compensatory increases in hematopoiesis are achieved by an expansion of active hematopoietic tissue into areas of the marrow that normally are inactive.

Components of the Marrow

The hematopoietic cells are arranged as cords of tissue that reside in a complex microenvironment composed of bone-lining cells, endothelial cells, macrophages, and T lymphocytes that are compartmentalized by branched, anastomosing trabeculae of bone. The microenvironment produces local factors, CSFs, that influence the cell line toward which a multipotential stem cell will differentiate. The microenvironment also has a role in differentiation and proliferation of hematopoietic stem cells. About 50% of the volume of the medullary cavity is fat and 50% is occupied by hematopoietic cells in middle-aged healthy adults of most species. Change in the number of hematopoietic cells is accompanied by a corresponding increase or decrease in the amount of fat.

Vasculature and Stroma

The marrow is supplied by arterioles derived primarily from nutrient arteries. Arterioles connect to venous sinuses, which drain into larger veins. Circulating blood remains within a closed vascular system and normally does not enter the hematopoietic cords. Delivery of marrow cells to the periphery takes place across the wall of the vascular sinus.

Fibroblastic cells are the main component of the marrow stroma, forming a meshwork that supports macrophages, hematopoietic cells, and other free cells and providing diverse hematopoietic microenvironments.

Hematopoietic Cells

Stem cells and their committed and differentiating progeny make up the hematopoietic portion of the marrow. Macrophages in the marrow store iron for release to developing erythroid cells, and phagocytize particulate matter and damaged cells. Lymphoid precursors are derived from the pluripotential hematopoietic stem cell, but differentiation and most cell division take place in lymphoid tissues (lymph nodes, spleen, and thymus). Lymphocytes make up <10% of normal marrow cells and are probably part of the recirculating lymphocyte pool.

Pluripotential hematopoietic stem cells consist of a finite number of cells capable of self-renewal as well as differentiation, so the number of stem cells cannot increase but remains constant through life unless they are destroyed by some disease mechanism. Morphologically, stem cells are poorly characterized mesenchymal cells that resemble small lymphocytes. They are named by their behavior in culture systems. The spleen colony-forming unit (CFU-S) cell is the most immature cell and gives rise to precursors capable of forming any blood cells (multilineage progenitor cells). The existence of the CFU-S was proved when syngeneic marrow was transplanted to mice whose hematopoietic system was destroyed by radiation. Discrete colonies of hematopoietic cells developed in the spleens and marrow of treated mice. Individual colonies differentiated in vitro into all of the hematopoietic cell lines. When these colonies were examined at various times during culture, they were found to have mixed populations of cells; thus, a single cell can give rise to all cell lines. The earliest division appears to be between lymphoid and nonlymphoid progenitors. Replication of progenitors occurs in response to signals from hematopoietic growth factors. Those affecting the earliest stem cells are less specific and include interleukin (IL-3) and granulocyte-monocyte CSF (GM-CSF). As progenitor cells replicate and become committed to one cell line, their morphology evolves to the point when they become recognizable on cytological evaluation of the marrow. In the normal marrow, a few early precursors (blasts) of each cell line are seen with progressively larger numbers of more mature cells (**Part B**). These precursors respond to more specific growth factors such as granulocyte CSF (G-CSF), erythropoietin, and thrombopoietin that move resting cells into mitosis as well as shorten the maturation time. These precursors continue to divide and mature. Most eventually mature to the point where cell division stops, but maturation continues for a time in the marrow. Certain mature cells may even be stored for a time, but all are eventually released and enter the circulation either to function there or to travel to tissues.

Production and Differentiation

Red Blood Cell Production

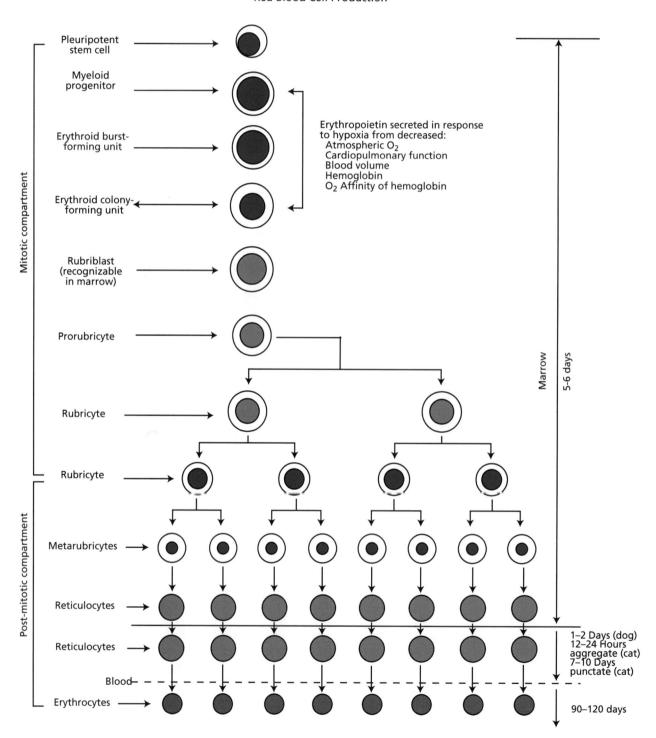

Pleuripotent stem cell

Myeloid progenitor

Erythroid burst-forming unit

Erythroid colony-forming unit

Erythropoietin secreted in response to hypoxia from decreased:
Atmospheric O_2
Cardiopulmonary function
Blood volume
Hemoglobin
O_2 Affinity of hemoglobin

Rubriblast (recognizable in marrow)

Prorubricyte

Rubricyte

Rubricyte

Metarubricytes

Reticulocytes

Reticulocytes

Blood

Erythrocytes

Mitotic compartment

Post-mitotic compartment

Marrow

5-6 days

1–2 Days (dog)
12–24 Hours aggregate (cat)
7–10 Days punctate (cat)

90–120 days

In order for an animal to survive, a constant source of oxygen must be available to the tissues. Normal red cells are efficient in taking up oxygen as it diffuses from the alveoli of the lungs through the endothelium and the red cell membrane to bind with hemoglobin. Oxygen must then be released by hemoglobin and pass through the vasculature into peripheral tissues. If too few red cells are present, as in anemia, oxygen delivery will be decreased. If too many red cells are present, the viscosity of the blood will be too high for adequate circulation through the small peripheral capillaries. The stimulus for increased production of red blood cells by the marrow is a decrease in oxygen tension in the blood, and more precisely in the kidney. Healthy individuals may have decreased oxygen tension because of decreased atmospheric oxygen, as would occur during travel at high altitudes. It may also occur in patients with pulmonary insufficiency, or heart failure.

Erythropoietin

The stimulating growth factor for red blood cells is erythropoietin (EPO), which is produced in the vascular endothelium of the kidney (**Figure**). In most species, EPO, a glycoprotein hormone, is produced solely in the kidneys, but in some species, a minor amount also is produced by the liver. If the kidneys are normal, the concentration of EPO increases in the blood whenever hypoxia occurs. Usually hypoxia is generalized, but interference with renal arterial blood flow might also be interpreted by the kidneys as a need for increased EPO production. EPO was the first of the hematopoietic growth factors to be identified, and (for human EPO) to be cloned and produced for clinical use. EPO increases the production of rubriblasts primarily by stimulating relatively mature progenitors (erythroid colony-forming units, CFU-Es), and in severe anemia or hypoxia, very high concentrations of EPO also will stimulate the more immature progenitors (erythroid burst-forming units, BFU-Es) and cause multilineage progenitor cells to commit to becoming erythroid progenitors (see **Figure**). The advantage of initially stimulating the more mature progenitors is that the process is more efficient to meet the day-to-day needs for new red cells, because it does not have to start over at the most immature progenitor. The CFU-Es are the immediate precursors of the rubriblasts, the earliest morphologically recognizable red cell precursors. The marrow transit time for developing erythrocytes is decreased as concentrations of EPO increase, causing some mitotic divisions to be skipped and the nucleus to be extruded prematurely. When this happens, young enucleated, but not fully mature red cells (reticulocytes) are released from the marrow (*see* Chapter 4). Most importantly, when an increased need for red cells occurs, EPO stimulates output *primarily* by increasing stem cell and committed progenitor cell input rather than by shortening the maturation time. Whenever the concentration of EPO increases, the marrow increases the rate of red cell production to 5–10 times the usual rate, depending on the severity of the need. Other hormones that potentiate the effects of EPO are thyroid hormones and androgens; estrogen and by-products of chronic inflammation act to suppress erythropoiesis.

Since EPO is produced in the kidneys, it is logical that patients with chronic renal failure can become severely anemic (*see* Chapter 23). Recombinant human EPO has essentially eliminated the need for transfusions in human patients with renal failure, and has been used with some success in dogs and cats.

Chronic hypoxia and certain renal lesions may result in too much EPO, which then causes too many red cells to be produced. *Polycythemia vera* is a chronic malignancy in which the bone marrow continues to produce red cells even when a decrease in EPO tells it to stop. In all of the above-mentioned conditions, the red cell count can become so high that the viscosity of the blood increases to the point that heart failure occurs. (*See* Chapter 28.)

Red Cell Production

Approximately 1% of circulating red cells are replaced daily, depending on the life span of red cells in each species. Generally, the smaller the animal, the shorter the life span of the red cells. This may be related to the more rapid metabolism and circulation time in smaller animals. Life span may be limited by the number of times the cell must travel through the spleen.

As new cells differentiate from a rubriblast to a mature red cell over 5–6 days, several morphological and metabolic changes occur (see **Figure**). As cytoplasmic RNA levels decrease and hemoglobin is formed, the cytoplasm of maturing red cell precursors changes from a deep blue to a pink-orange as seen with Wright's stain of a bone marrow aspirate. This color is first noticeable at the rubricyte stage. Hemoglobin production is completed at the reticulocyte stage. Iron, necessary for heme formation, is delivered bound to transferrin, which attaches to transmembrane receptors on erythroid precursors. With each mitosis, the cells become smaller. The rubricyte is the most mature red cell precursor that retains the ability to divide as part of the mitotic compartment. The metarubricyte, which can only mature, has a small blue-black homogeneous nonfunctional nucleus that, in mammals, is usually extruded in the marrow, leaving a reticulocyte, a slightly larger and more basophilic cell than a mature red cell. Sometimes a small fragment of nuclear material, called a *Howell-Jolly body*, is left in the mature red cell. Usually this is removed by the spleen, so the number of Howell-Jolly bodies is sometimes increased in patients with nonfunctional spleens or those from whom the spleen has been removed surgically.

Even in species such as birds, reptiles, amphibians, and fish, in which mature red cells retain the nucleus, it becomes nonfunctional and mature red cells cannot divide. Mammals are said to have an advantage because enucleated red cells are more flexible and better able to navigate small capillaries; however, species with nucleated red cells seem to function well despite their phylogenetically inferior cells.

The developing red cells lose their mitochondria, RNA, and thus their ability to make new protein. The resulting cell is suited perfectly for its function of oxygen delivery.

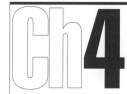 **Reticulocytes**

A   Reticulocytes

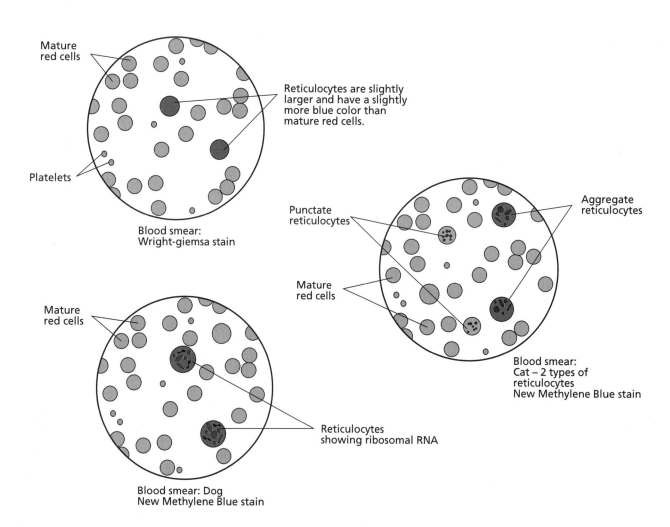

Mature red cells

Reticulocytes are slightly larger and have a slightly more blue color than mature red cells.

Platelets

Blood smear:
Wright-giemsa stain

Punctate reticulocytes

Aggregate reticulocytes

Mature red cells

Blood smear:
Cat – 2 types of reticulocytes
New Methylene Blue stain

Mature red cells

Reticulocytes showing ribosomal RNA

Blood smear: Dog
New Methylene Blue stain

B   **Correction of Reticulocyte Count for the Degree of Anemia**

Corrections can be done in either of two ways:

1) Absolute reticulocyte count/ml= Observed reticulocyte percentage x Red blood cell count /ml

2) Corrected reticulocyte percentage = Observed reticulocyte percentage x $\dfrac{\text{Patient's Hct}}{\text{Normal Hct}}$;

* Note: 45% is used for normal dog reticulocyte percentage; 37% is used for cats

EXAMPLE: An anemic dog has a red blood cell count of $3.4 \times 10^{6}/\mu l$,
an Hct of 25% with an observed reticulocyte percentage of 9%

1) Absolute reticulocyte count = 9% of 3.4×10^{6} = 306,000/μl
This is greater than 60,000/μl so the anemia is regenerative

2) Corrected reticulocyte percentage = 9% x $\dfrac{25\%}{45\%}$ = 5%
This is greater than 1% so the anemia is regenerative

Reticulocytes are immature enucleated erythroid cells with considerable quantities of ribosomal and mitochondrial RNA. They are slightly larger than mature red cells (**Part A**). With a Romanowsky stain such as Wright's or Wright-Giemsa, the RNA dissolves during alcohol fixation, giving a uniform blue-gray color (polychromasia) to the cells (see **Part A**). When these polychromatophilic red cells are stained with new methylene blue, the RNA precipitates, forming dark blue-purple granules in the cytoplasm. While a subjective evaluation of red cell production may be made on the basis of polychromasia and increased size as indicated by the mean corpuscular volume (MCV), the reticulocyte count is the most useful and accurate method of quantitating marrow erythroid activity. Most reticulocytes remain in the bone marrow until they are mature erythrocytes. Under the influence of erythropoietin they may be released early. After acute blood loss or hemolysis, reticulocytes will increase in the blood only after 3–4 days.

In severe acute regenerative anemias, nucleated red cells, usually metarubricytes, may enter the blood along with reticulocytes. The appearance of nucleated red cells in the blood without reticulocytes is an inappropriate response and is *not* a sign of regeneration.

When a reticulocyte count is done, smears are made and stained with new methylene blue. The number of reticulocytes counted is reported as a percentage of total red cells. This percentage can be multiplied by the red cell count to calculate the number of reticulocytes per microliter of blood.

Interpretation of Reticulocyte Count

If blood loss or red cell destruction were fully compensated by an increased production of red cells, it would be possible to maintain a normal Hct and a high reticulocyte count (reticulocytosis). In fact, a high MCV, polychromasia, and reticulocytosis may be the first indications of low-grade blood loss or hemolysis.

As an example, the normal canine reticulocyte number is about 60,000/µL (1% of the circulating red cells). If the Hct (and red cell count) falls by half but red cell production is constant, the reticulocyte percentage nevertheless will still be 1%, but the absolute count will be only 30,000/µL. Any anemic animal with <1% of reticulocytes, or with an absolute count of <60,000/µL, would be considered to have a nonregenerative anemia. No further calculations would be needed to reach that conclusion. To say that an anemia is regenerative, the output of reticulocytes should be greater than the baseline rate. If the absolute number of reticulocytes is >60,000/µL, or if the corrected reticulocyte count is >1%, the anemia is likely to be regenerative (**Part B**).

An additional correction (Reticulocyte Production Index, RPI) is sometimes made for prolonged reticulocyte maturation time in severe anemia. This implies that the more severe the anemia, the greater the marrow response should be before the anemia is considered to be regenerative. The RPI has been validated as a useful indicator of regeneration in humans but most veterinary hematologists use only the corrected reticulocyte percentage or absolute reticulocyte count in animals. However, it is probably true in general that a greater number of reticulocytes should be present in animals with severe anemia compared to those with mild anemia for one to be confident that an adequate marrow response is present.

Cats

Cats are unique in that they have 2 types of reticulocytes. The most immature are aggregate reticulocytes, which have many coarse granules. The more mature are punctate reticulocytes, which have a few fine granules. The aggregate reticulocytes mature in 12–24 hours like those of the dog and are an indicator of recent marrow activity. Most laboratories report only the aggregate count, which is "corrected for the Hct" or used to calculate the absolute count. Only aggregate reticulocytes have enough RNA to cause them to be polychromatophilic on routinely stained smears. After a single severe episode of bleeding or hemolysis, aggregate reticulocytes appear in peripheral blood after 2–3 days, with a peak at about 4 days, and drop back to ≤1% by the 8th day. Punctate reticulocytes begin to increase in number on about the 4th day and continue to increase before returning to normal after the Hct has reached a normal value on about the 12th–14th day. It appears that in mild anemia, only punctate reticulocytes are released from marrow and may persist in the blood for 10–12 days. Normal reticulocyte counts in the cat are 0.5%–1.0% for aggregate and 1.5%–10.5% for punctate.

Ruminants

Healthy cattle and sheep do not have circulating reticulocytes. In anemic animals, reticulocytes are released in proportion to the degree of anemia, and basophilic stippling is seen. In some cattle with chronic anemia reticulocytosis may not be present in the blood, but erythroid hyperplasia and reticulocytosis are present in the marrow.

Horses

Even in severely anemic horses, reticulocytes rarely are released from marrow to circulate in blood; therefore, reticulocyte counts are not done on horse blood. The response to anemia in the horse is assessed by examining the marrow for erythroid hyperplasia, or by evaluating the MCV, as macrocytosis may be an indicator of increased marrow activity.

Marrow Changes in Regenerative Anemia

Examination of the marrow is not needed if significant reticulocytosis is present. In some situations, erythroid hyperplasia may occur in the marrow without reticulocytosis. There are 2 possible explanations for this: 1) it takes 3–4 days to mount a reticulocyte response after acute blood loss; 2) intramedullary destruction of red cells may occur, as in immune-mediated hemolysis where even red cell precursors may be destroyed.

Ch5 Structure and Metabolism

A Composition of the Red Blood Cell Membrane

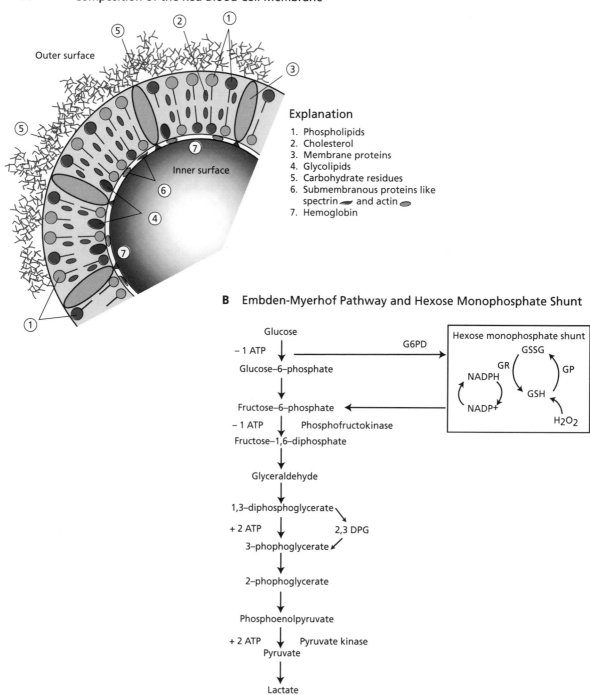

Outer surface

Inner surface

Explanation

1. Phospholipids
2. Cholesterol
3. Membrane proteins
4. Glycolipids
5. Carbohydrate residues
6. Submembranous proteins like spectrin and actin
7. Hemoglobin

B Embden-Myerhof Pathway and Hexose Monophosphate Shunt

Glucose

− 1 ATP

Glucose–6–phosphate

G6PD

Hexose monophosphate shunt

GSSG

GR

NADPH

GP

GSH

NADP+

H_2O_2

Fructose–6–phosphate

− 1 ATP   Phosphofructokinase

Fructose–1,6–diphosphate

Glyceraldehyde

1,3–diphosphoglycerate

+ 2 ATP

2,3 DPG

3–phophoglycerate

2–phophoglycerate

Phosphoenolpyruvate

+ 2 ATP   Pyruvate kinase

Pyruvate

Lactate

GSSG=oxidized glutathione; GSH=reduced glutathione; GR=glutathione reductase; GP=glutothione peroxidase;
NADPH=reduced nicotinamide-adenine dinucleotide phosphate; NADP=nicotinamide-adenine dinucleotide phosphate;
ATP=adenosine triphosphate; G6PD=glucose-6-phosphate dehydrogenase; DPG=diphosphoglycerate

The mature mammalian red cell has disposed of its nucleus, ribosomes, and mitochondria. Its biconcave shape with a high surface area–volume ratio is well suited for oxygen uptake and delivery and movement at rapid speeds through the microcirculation. During a life span of 3–4 months, a red cell may make a half-million round-trips and travel about 300 miles. Cells can change shape to traverse small vessels and sinusoids. Since red cells are dense, they travel in the center of large vessels. In the presence of large macromolecules such as fibrinogen, red cells may travel stacked, in arrangements called *rouleaux*, like small dishes held together by weak surface-bridging forces. The lighter monocytes, neutrophils, and platelets roll along the endothelial surface, allowing them to stick, leave the circulation, and perform their respective functions when the need arises.

Species Variation

Mammalian red cells may display some variation on the theme of the biconcave disk, seen on blood smears as an area of central pallor surrounded by a pink-red outer area. Typical biconcave red cells are present in the dog, cow, and sheep. The mouse, cat, and goat have more flattened cells with slight concavity, seen on blood smears as a more uniform color with minimal to no central pallor. Other normal species variations include elliptical red cells in the camel, alpaca, and llama. Some species of deer have sickle-shaped cells that function normally.

Red Cell Membrane and Cytoskeleton

The membrane, composed of proteins (48%), lipids (44%), and carbohydrates (8%), is essential for deformability and resilience of the cells (**Part A**). The carbohydrates are in the form of glycoproteins or glycolipids. The membrane lipids play the major role in cell shape and surface area. Permeability to certain cations is necessary to maintain the proper ionic gradient inside and outside of the cell. The lipids, primarily cholesterol and phospholipids, are arranged in a bilayer in which the membrane proteins are embedded. Changes in membrane phospholipid and cholesterol composition occur with liver disease and may be seen on a blood smear as target cells. The glycolipids in the outer aspect of the bilayer confer a negative charge (zeta potential) and make up the blood group antigens (*see* Chapter 15). The zeta potential keeps red cells from agglutinating under normal circumstances.

Plasma proteins are responsible for the movement of electrolytes, particularly sodium and potassium in and out of the red cell. Species differences exist, however; horses, cattle, humans, and some breeds of dogs have low concentrations of sodium and high concentrations of potassium in red cells, whereas most dogs and cats have low concentrations of potassium. The active exchange of sodium and potassium is controlled by a pump fueled by ATP.

Beneath the membrane is a cytoskeleton of structural proteins that determine the shape of the cell. Spectrin, unique to red cells, is a long, flexible protein that forms an elastic network that lines the inner surface of the membrane. Spectrin is linked to the membrane by membrane proteins, ankyrin and band 4.1 (named for its location on gel electrophoresis of the membrane). Actin is another cytoskeletal protein that plays a key role in maintaining cell shape.

Metabolism

The mature red cell depends almost entirely on the Embden-Meyerhof pathway for energy (**Part B**). The long life span of the red cell is ensured through 2 general mechanisms: production of ATP for energy, and defense against oxidation via the pentose phosphate pathway. Red cells utilize anaerobic glycolysis despite the fact that large quantities of oxygen are present in the hemoglobin of the cell. Red cells are rich in 2,3-diphosphoglycerate (2,3-DPG), formed by the Rapoport-Luebering pathway. The primary function of 2,3-DPG is to facilitate unloading of oxygen. Ordinarily the oxygen is picked up and delivered by the red cell without undergoing any changes; it is simply cargo. Occasionally an oxygen molecule will be converted to more reactive species such as superoxide (O_2^-) or hydrogen peroxide (H_2O_2). These compounds must be removed for the red cell to survive. Protective substances within the cell include superoxide dismutase, which converts O_2^- to H_2O_2 and oxygen. Catalase then converts H_2O_2 to oxygen and water. The most important protective system, however, is the glutathione antioxidant system contained in the hexose monophosphate pathway.

In this system, glutathione reacts with hydrogen peroxide catalyzed by glutathione peroxidase to oxidized glutathione. The oxidized glutathione is then converted back to reduced glutathione by reduced nicotinamide-adenine dinucleotide phosphate (NADPH) catalyzed by glutathione reductase.

Thus, the system cycles between the reduced and oxidized forms, converting 1 molecule of hydrogen peroxide to water in each cycle. Because NADPH is consumed, this reducing agent must be regenerated utilizing the glucose-6-phosphate dehydrogenase (G6PD) reaction.

In normal animals, the hexose monophosphate pathway functions minimally. It can increase its activity rapidly when oxidized substrates accumulate. The hexose monophosphate pathway is impaired in humans with a hereditary deficiency of G6PD. This defect has not been described in domestic animals; however, oxidative damage to red cells occurs through acquired disorders, especially those caused by toxins (*see* Chapter 18).

Oxidants cause damage to hemoglobin and to the red cell membrane, resulting in methemoglobinemia, denaturation of hemoglobin seen as Heinz bodies, and hemolysis.

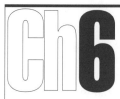

Hemoglobin and Oxygen Transport

Hemoglobin Structure and Function

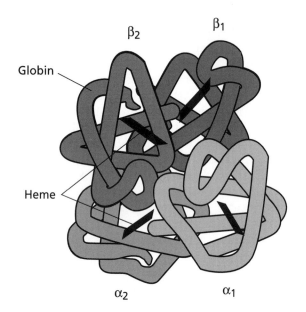

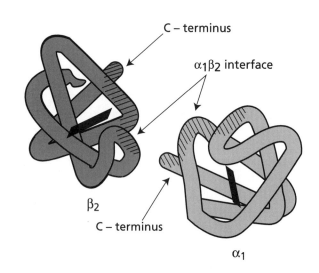

B O_2 Dissociation Curve

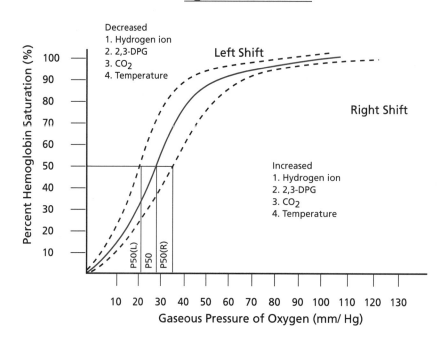

Structure of Hemoglobin

Hemoglobin is an oxygen-transporting protein with a molecular size of about 65,000 d. It makes up about a third of the total weight and 95% of the dry weight of the red cell. Each tetrameric molecule consists of 4 heme units, each with a covalently bound polypeptide globin chain, 2 α and 2 β chains. Two αβ dimers combine to form the complete hemoglobin molecule (**Part A**).

Heme is a large flat disk consisting of protoporphyrin plus iron. The iron must remain in the reduced (ferrous) state. Heme is synthesized in the mitochondria of rubricytes and metarubricytes and to a lesser extent in reticulocytes. The basic structure of heme appears fixed, and interspecies differences are not seen.

Globin chains are synthesized on polyribosomes in the cytoplasm by genetic information carried by messenger RNA. Each heme group is attached to a globin chain by linkage of iron to a histidine residue. These histidines are situated so that hemoglobin can bind to oxygen reversibly. The 2 regions where the 2 αβ dimers come in contact are known as the $\alpha_1\beta_2$ interfaces where oxygen binding and release take place. Differences in the amino acid sequence of globin are responsible for differences between species, and between adult and fetal hemoglobin. For example, cat hemoglobin has 8 reactive sulfhydryl groups, compared to 2–4 in most other mammals. Fetal hemoglobin has a higher affinity for oxygen, which provides improved extraction of oxygen from the maternal circulation to that of the fetus. In spite of this, there has been no observable disadvantage to fetal oxygenation in species such as dogs and horses lacking fetal hemoglobin.

Function of Hemoglobin

Hemoglobin binds oxygen reversibly in the lungs. It must take up as much as possible to become fully saturated. The oxygen-binding site is the iron of the heme group. The iron normally stays in the ferrous (2+) form during oxygen uptake, transport, and delivery. In the tissues the oxygen is unloaded, as much as is needed to support life.

To accomplish this, oxygen binds to hemoglobin in a cooperative fashion. Thus, the uptake of 1 oxygen molecule will facilitate the uptake of the next. This can occur because the hemoglobin molecule can exist in 2 conformations. The T (taut) state is characterized by a close fit between the 2 $\alpha_1\beta_2$ regions and has a relatively low oxygen affinity. The R (relaxed) state has a wider separation between the $\alpha_1\beta_2$ regions and a higher oxygen affinity. As oxygen is taken up, the molecule favors the R state; when it is fully saturated and some is released, it changes toward the T state, lowering the affinity further and allowing the release of more oxygen. One measure of oxygen affinity is P_{50} (the partial pressure of oxygen, in millimeters of mercury, required for 50% saturation of hemoglobin). If the P_{50} is increased, the oxygen affinity is decreased.

This relationship between oxygen tension and saturation of the hemoglobin molecule with oxygen is expressed as an S-shaped or sigmoidal curve (**Part B**). This curve has great physiological importance as it shows that large amounts of oxygen can be bound or released with only small variations in oxygen tension.

Regulation of Oxygen Affinity

The ability of hemoglobin to alter its affinity for oxygen allows a person or animal to adapt to various environmental, physiological, or pathological situations.

The Bohr Effect

A fall in pH of the blood leads to a decrease in oxygen affinity of hemoglobin. Because pH in actively metabolizing tissues is lower than in the lungs, oxygen is unloaded in the tissues where it is needed. Then the red cell returns to the lungs, where the higher pH facilitates the uptake of more oxygen.

2,3-DPG

The red cell depends on anaerobic glycolysis for the production of 2,3-DPG, which binds to the β chains, stabilizing the T state and increasing the release of oxygen. Levels of 2,3-DPG rise under conditions of hypoxia and anemia. Unlike changes in pH, the changes in 2,3-DPG take place over hours. Both of these situations are more likely to occur in the tissues than in the lungs and are related to ongoing metabolic processes. Concentrations of 2,3-DPG rise in alkalosis and fall in acidosis, thus providing a counterbalance with the Bohr effect. Respiratory hyperventilation and alkalosis may be 1 mechanism by which 2,3-DPG increases in hypoxia and anemia. The levels of 2,3-DPG also rise when serum phosphate is increased. Renal failure often is accompanied by hyperphosphatemia and subsequently by anemia, but increased 2,3-DPG improves tissue oxygenation. The oxygen dissociation also shifts to favor oxygen unloading in situations of increased carbon dioxide and increased temperature. In some species such as cattle and cats, the chloride ion functions in the same manner as 2,3-DPG so that they do not depend on 2,3-DPG for tissue oxygenation.

In humans, a variety of abnormal hemoglobin variants have been identified. Genetic disorders such as thalassemia and sickle cell anemia are caused by variations in the amino acids comprising the globin chains. In sickle cell disease, aggregation of the hemoglobin molecules causes shape changes and rigidity of the red cells, resulting in occlusion of the capillaries and hemolysis. In thalassemias, defective synthesis of 1 or more polypeptide chains of the globin molecule occurs, resulting in hemolysis.

The only hemoglobinopathy recognized in domestic animals is porphyria. Erythropoietic porphyria occurs primarily in cattle but has been found rarely in cats and swine. Affected animals have a reddish brown discoloration of teeth, bones, and urine from an accumulation of these abnormal porphyrins, mild hemolysis may occur. In cattle, accumulation of these abnormal porphyrins in the skin causes a photosensitization reaction in white or nonpigmented areas of the skin and a sunburn reaction (*see* Chapter 20).

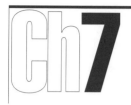

Destruction of Red Cells

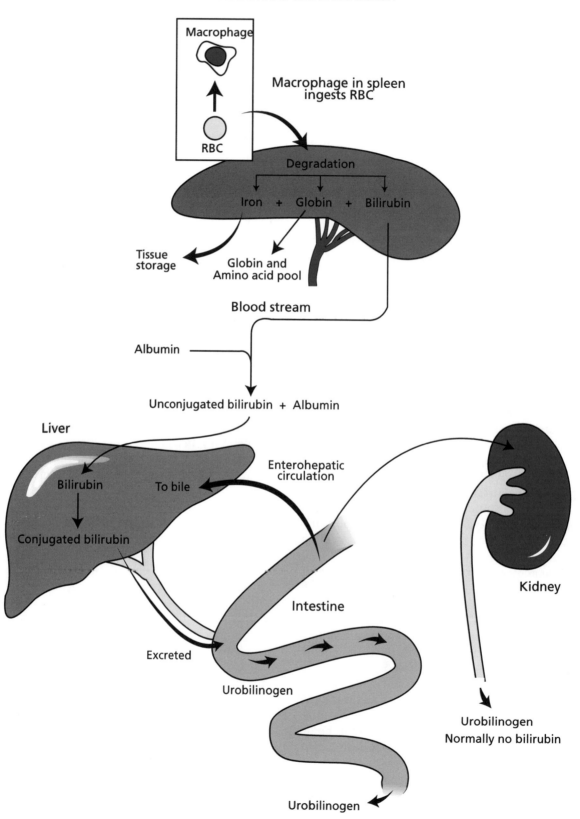

Red Blood Cell Destruction

Macrophage

RBC

Macrophage in spleen
ingests RBC

Degradation

Iron + Globin + Bilirubin

Tissue
storage

Globin and
Amino acid pool

Blood stream

Albumin

Unconjugated bilirubin + Albumin

Liver

Bilirubin

To bile

Conjugated bilirubin

Enterohepatic
circulation

Kidney

Excreted

Urobilinogen

Intestine

Urobilinogen
Normally no bilirubin

Urobilinogen

The normal life span of red cells is predetermined for each species. In smaller animals with a high metabolic rate, the survival time is shorter than in larger animals (*see* Chapter 3). An interesting exception is that of hibernating animals in which metabolism is suspended. For example, in the nonhibernating woodchuck, red cells live about 36 days. This survival time increases to about 112 days during hibernation.

On average, approximately 60,000 (1%) of the 6 million red cells per microliter in circulation are replaced daily. As cells age, several changes occur that increase the risk of removal from the circulation, primarily in the spleen. Red cells are normally deformable so that they can navigate small capillaries. Older cells become more rigid. A decrease in the ratio of surface area to volume due to osmotic swelling, loss of membrane, or fragmentation results in loss of the biconcave shape. Adequate ATP is required for maintenance of ionic and osmotic equilibrium. Hypoxia, acidosis, excessive intracellular calcium, and decreased ATP can reduce red cell deformability. The most decisive change that predisposes red cells to demise is a stiffening of hemoglobin-spectrin cross-linkages.

Natural IgG antibodies to neoantigens created during senescence make cells expressing these more attractive to mononuclear phagocytes. It has been hypothesized that modifications of the red cell membrane occur over time, perhaps exposing parts to which autoantibodies bind and facilitate removal by macrophages.

Role of the Spleen

The spleen is the main site for both normal and abnormal removal of red cells (**Figure**). Arteries enter the spleen from the capsule and pass through sinuses containing primarily red cells and are surrounded by lymphocytes (white pulp) (*see* Chapter 40). Some blood passes briskly through these sinuses and empties into veins. Other blood percolates through cords of loosely organized masses of mononuclear phagocytes and fibrous tissues before entering the venous circulation. It is in the cords with decreased oxygen tension, low pH, and hypoxia where old or abnormal red cells might be trapped and attacked by hungry phagocytes.

Most of the components of the red cell including the globin portion of hemoglobin are degraded into amino acids that are recycled into other proteins. Heme, however, is disposed of, with only the iron saved for reuse or storage. An understanding of the degradation of heme is important as excessive accumulation of certain intermediate substances provides clues toward recognition of the presence and possible causes of hemolysis in certain anemic patients (*see* Chapter 13).

The porphyrin ring is cleaved; the reaction is catalyzed by the microsomal enzyme heme oxygenase, producing iron and a tetrapyrrole biliverdin. The iron is transported bound to transferrin for incorporation into red cells or for storage. Biliverdin is reduced to bilirubin, which is released from the phagocyte into the circulation.

In the absence of a spleen, removal of old or defective red cells is impaired. Abnormal or misshapen red cells may be seen in the circulation. Some may contain nuclear remnants (Howell-Jolly bodies) or denatured hemoglobin (Heinz bodies) or even red cell parasites that normally would be removed by the spleen. Overall, the red cell life span remains the same in the absence of the spleen, probably because the mononuclear phagocytes of the liver and other organs work overtime to fulfill the role of those of the spleen.

Role of the Liver

Bound to albumin, bilirubin is transported to the liver. In the liver, the bilirubin is dissociated from albumin and enters the hepatocyte, where it is conjugated with uridine diphosphoglucuronide to form bilirubin-diglucuronide. The conjugated (water-soluble) bilirubin is excreted through the bile canaliculi into the intestine. In the intestine, some of the bilirubin is transformed by bacteria to a further reduced urobilinogen. Some of the urobilinogen is absorbed through the intestine. Most is reexcreted in the bile via the enterohepatic circulation and is excreted in feces, but some urobilinogen is normally excreted by the kidneys into the urine.

If any free hemoglobin enters the bloodstream through leakage either from phagocytes or from disease conditions causing rupture of red cells in the circulation, the free hemoglobin in the plasma (hemoglobinemia) binds to a plasma protein, haptoglobin, and is rapidly transported to the liver where the hemoglobin is degraded as it would have been in the phagocytes. When breakdown (hemolysis) of red cells occurs beyond the capacity of haptoglobin to bind it, the excess hemoglobin is excreted in the urine (hemoglobinuria).

In the presence of hemolysis regardless of the cause, evidence of increased heme breakdown includes jaundice (icterus), a yellow color of the skin, scleras, and mucous membranes, and increased concentrations of bilirubin, which can be measured in the serum. The concentration of conjugated bilirubin is measured directly and thus called *direct bilirubin*. The concentration of unconjugated bilirubin is measured indirectly by subtracting the amount of conjugated bilirubin from the total amount. Thus, the unconjugated bilirubin is called *indirect bilirubin*. If the liver is normal, hemolysis can cause an increase primarily in unconjugated bilirubin, since the liver can conjugate and excrete it as it arrives. In the presence of liver disease or biliary obstruction, an increase in conjugated bilirubin occurs. It can leak from hepatocytes or build up when canaliculi are swollen (intrahepatic obstruction) or when the bile duct is obstructed, as might occur with stones, tumors, or pancreatic disease (extrahepatic obstruction). In real life, however, these distinctions are rarely clear-cut, and increases in both conjugated and unconjugated bilirubin may occur with hemolysis and with liver disease.

Products of bilirubin metabolism, urobilinogen and conjugated bilirubin, also may be excreted in the urine if their concentrations in the blood are excessive. Unconjugated bilirubin never occurs in the urine since it is insoluble in water.

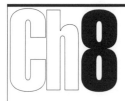

Evaluation of Erythrocytes

A The Complete Blood Count

1. White blood cell count (WBC count)
2. Red blood cell count (RBC count)
3. Hematocrit (Hct) packed cell volume (PCV)
4. Hemoglobin concentration (Hb)
5. Red cell indices, mean corpuscular volume, mean corpuscular hemoglobin, and mean corpuscular hemoglobin concentration (MCV, MCH, and MCHC)
6. Platelet count depending on species
7. Red cell distribution width (RDW)
8. Mean platelet volume (MPV)
9. Evaluation of peripheral blood smear
   a. Differential WBC count
   b. Estimation of platelet number
   c. Evaluation of cell morphology of presence of inclusions
   d. Evaluation for blood parasites or other organisms

B Morphologic Descriptions of Red Blood Cells

Acanthocytes: erythrocytes in which the cell membrane contains increased cholesterol levels which cause spike-like projections. These are seen in animals with liver disease.
Anisocytosis: variation (heterogeneity) of erythrocyte size
Basophilic stippling: Fine bluish inclusions scattered throughtout the cytoplasm of the erythrocyte
Elliptocytes: oval or elliptical erythrocytes
Heinz bodies: hemoglobin precipitates visible in fresh blood as shown by phase microscopy or by supravital staining
Howell-Jolly bodies: Chromatin residues in erythrocytes
Hypochromia: erythrocytes with decreased hemoglobin content and decreased staining intensity
Leptocyte (target cells): cells with "Mexican hat" or "bull's-eye" appearance
Macrocytosis: erythrocytes with increased volume and diameter
Microcytosis: erythrocytes with decreased volume and diameter
Normochromia: normal color intensity on a Romanowsky stain
Normocytes: erythrocytes that are normal size and shape
Poikilocytosis: variation of erythrocyte shape on the blood film
Polychromasia: variation of sataining color of erythrocytes on the same blood film (cells that stain bluish or purple represent reticulocytes)
Schistocytes: fragmented erythrocytes of varied size and shape (usually angular in appearance)
Spherocytes (dogs only): small erythrocytes of spherical shape and lacking normal central pallor (homogeneous staining of cells)

C Comparison of Morphologic and Etiologic Classification of Anemia

Morphologic Classification	Etiologic Classification
Normocytic normochromic (Normal MCV, MCHC)	Depression of erythrogenesis Chronic inflammation Chronic renal insufficiency Endocrine deficiencies Neoplasia Marrow hypoplasia Acute hemorrhage (first 1 – 3 days) Feline leukemia virus infection
Macrocytic normochromic (Increased MCV, normal MCHC)	Dietary deficiencies Poodle macrocytosis (healthy miniature poodles, no anemia) Feline leukemia virus infection Regenerative anemias
Macrocytic hypochromic (Increased MCV, low MCHC)	Regenerative anemias
Microcytic normochromic/ hypochromic (Decreased MCV and normal or low MCHC)	Iron deficiency Congenital portosystemic shunts (may not be anemic)

D Red Cell Distibution Width (RDW)

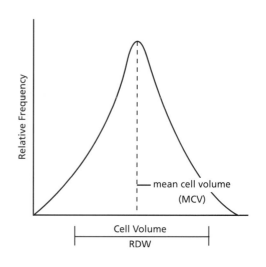

The Complete Blood Cell Count

When a complete blood cell count (CBC), sometimes called the *hemogram*, is performed, the numbers, size, and morphology of red (RBC) and white blood cells (WBC) and platelets are evaluated. The parameters measured for the standard CBC are listed in **Parts A** and **B**.

Blood is collected from a peripheral vein and placed in a purple-top tube that contains EDTA, which tightly binds calcium, making it unavailable for coagulation. Blood smears should be made within 2–3 hours after specimen collection, to avoid degenerative changes in cell morphology. If blood is refrigerated, cell counts remain stable for approximately 24 hours. In this chapter, evaluation of erythrocytes is addressed. Issues of white cells and platelets are discussed in Chapters 29 and 42.

RBC Count, Expressed as $10^6/\mu L$

Cell counts can be performed either manually or semi-automatically. An RBC count performed manually using a hemacytometer has a large degree of error (10%–20%) and is not worth the time and effort it takes to perform. If the instrument is properly calibrated for the species in question, electronic RBC counts are accurate.

In the impedance method, a diluted specimen of whole blood is introduced into a counting chamber. Cells are counted and sized based on the measurement of changes in electrical current that are produced by a particle passing through an aperture of known dimensions. As a cell passes a transitory increase in the resistance is measured as an electrical pulse, the magnitude of which is directly proportional to the size of the cell. The pulses are processed to yield cell count and size (volume) data, which typically are displayed as histograms and numerical values. These counters are particle counters that classify particles as erythrocytes, platelets, or different types of leukocytes based on cell volume.

Hct or Packed Cell Volume (PCV) Expressed as a Percentage

These two parameters represent the percentage of the volume of whole blood composed of red cells. The Hct is calculated using the measured mean corpuscular volume (MCV) and the RBC count. The PCV is determined by centrifuging blood in a microhematocrit capillary tube until red cells are packed at the bottom of the tube. Examination of the spun tube reveals three distinct strata: at the top, a clear fluid that is plasma; in the middle, a very thin layer called the buffy coat that consists of white cells, platelets, and reticulocytes; and the bottom layer of packed red cells. The percentage of the length of the entire column filled by red cells is the PCV. For practical purposes, the two terms *Hct* and *PCV* may be used interchangeably, although the PCV typically is 1%–2% higher than the Hct. The Hct is relatively constant between species, whereas the number and size of red cells are more variable.

The color of the plasma in the hematocrit tube should be noted. The plasma of normal dogs and cats is colorless to light yellow; that of horses and cows, medium yellow. If the plasma appears red, free hemoglobin (hemoglobinemia) is present, indicative of hemolysis that has occurred, either in vitro or in vivo. An intense yellow color indicates icterus due to hepatobiliary disease, hemolytic anemia, or both. If the plasma appears turbid, lipemia is the most likely cause. Lipemia can occur normally after eating, or if the patient has a metabolic disorder.

Hemoglobin Concentration (Hb), Expressed as gm/dL

Hemoglobin is measured by lysing a diluted suspension of red cells, reacting the lysate with ferrocyanide to produce cyanmethemoglobin, and spectrophotometrically determining the Hb. Since the measurement of Hb is by spectrophotometry, substances that increase the optical density of the solution will cause spuriously high readings. Lipemia and the presence of many Heinz bodies are 2 major causes of error in Hb measurement. The numerical value for Hb should be approximately one-third of the Hct; e.g., the normal dog Hb is 14 gm/dL, and the Hct is 42%. Factors that affect the measurement of 1 value but not the other will alter this relationship.

Red Cell Indices

Red cell indices are expressions of red cell size and Hb that are used to classify anemias. These indices usually are calculated from the Hct, Hb, and RBC count. Utilizing the indices one may be able to determine the cause of anemia, (*See* **Part C**).

The MCV expressed in femtoliters (fL-10^{15}L) is the volume of the average red cell as measured by hematology instruments. It can be calculated as MCV = (Hct/RBC) × 10. Of all of the indices, the MCV is the most useful in determining the cause of an anemia.

The mean corpuscular hemoglobin concentration (MCHC), expressed in gm/dL indicates the Hb in the average red cell and is a weight to volume relationship. It can be calculated as MCHC = (Hb/Hct) × 100 (**Part C**).

For all species, the MCHC should be 30–36 gm/dL. Because of the solubility of hemoglobin, a hyperchromic state is not possible. An MCHC >36 gm/dL indicates technical errors in measuring Hct or Hb, or both.

Sometimes an additional index, the mean corpuscular hemoglobin (MCH), expressed in picograms (pg), is reported. Calculated as MCH = (Hb/RBC) × 10, this indicates the amount of hemoglobin in the average red cell. The MCH does not provide additional information so is not often used in evaluating red cells.

Red Cell Distribution Width (RDW)

The RDW is a measure of the variability of erythrocyte size (anisocytosis). An increased RDW indicates the presence of a subpopulation of red cells larger or smaller (or both) than those represented by the MCV (**Part D**).

Anemia

A Changes in Packed Cell Volume (PCV) and Total Protein (TP) in Various Conditions

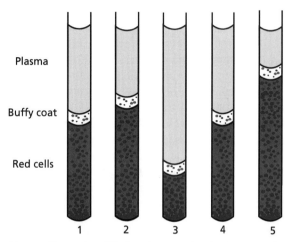

Plasma

Buffy coat

Red cells

1   2   3   4   5

Five capillary tubes filled to the same level with blood from animals with different problems (the PCV and TP levels are approximate and cannot be determined from the figures):

1. Normal PCV (30% – 45%), TP 6.0 – 7.5gm/dL.
2. Dehydration – loss of plasma with normal number of red cells. PCV appears higher than normal. If animal were rehydrated, the PCV would decrease to normal. PCV 60%, TP 8.5gm/dL.
3. Anemia – loss of red cells with normal plasma volume. PCV 20%, TP 7.0gm/dL.
4. Anemia and dehydration – loss of both red cells and plasma. Both PCV and TP appear higher than they are. This situation must be recognized by clinical examination of the patients. PCV 40%, TP 8.9gm/dL.
5. Polycythemia – increase in total red cell mass with normal plasma volume. PCV 75%, TP 6.8gm/dL.

B Relationship Between PCV and Plasma Protein

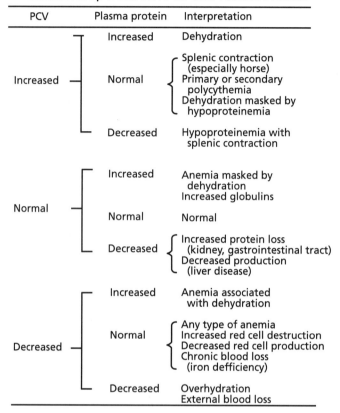

PCV	Plasma protein	Interpretation
Increased	Increased	Dehydration
	Normal	Splenic contraction (especially horse) Primary or secondary polycythemia Dehydration masked by hypoproteinemia
	Decreased	Hypoproteinemia with splenic contraction
Normal	Increased	Anemia masked by dehydration Increased globulins
	Normal	Normal
	Decreased	Increased protein loss (kidney, gastrointestinal tract) Decreased production (liver disease)
Decreased	Increased	Anemia associated with dehydration
	Normal	Any type of anemia Increased red cell destruction Decreased red cell production Chronic blood loss (iron defficiency)
	Decreased	Overhydration External blood loss

C   Approach to the Anemic Patient

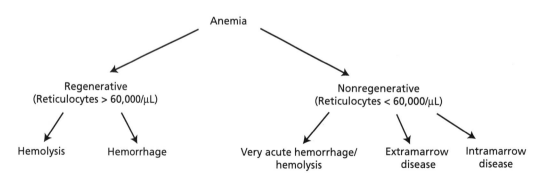

Anemia

Regenerative (Reticulocytes > 60,000/μL)

Hemolysis   Hemorrhage

Nonregenerative (Reticulocytes < 60,000/μL)

Very acute hemorrhage/ hemolysis   Extramarrow disease   Intramarrow disease

*A*nemia may be defined as a decrease in total red cell mass to a point where oxygen-carrying capacity of the blood is compromised. The normal response of the marrow to blood loss or destruction is increased production; as long as production keeps up, the red cell number remains normal and anemia is not present. When production fails to match losses, anemia results. This is seen as a below-normal total RBC count, Hb and Hct, or PCV. Two major causes of anemia are loss of red cells through bleeding or destruction (hemolysis) and decreased or abnormal production of red cells in the marrow. Thus, anemia should be considered a clinical sign rather than a diagnosis, and the cause must be sought before an appropriate treatment plan and prognosis can be formulated.

The red cell count and Hct must be interpreted in the light of other findings and the history. Measurements of these parameters by themselves may be misleading, because they represent relative numbers per unit of blood volume. In states of dehydration, the plasma volume may be decreased so the relative red cell mass may appear higher and thus mask the presence of anemia or may lead one to suspect polycythemia (increased red cell mass). The PCV can be measured with and compared to the total serum protein (TP) concentration. With dehydration, both the PCV and the TP increase, whereas in polycythemia only the PCV increases (**Parts A** and **B**).

Signs of Anemia

Clinical signs shown by an anemic animal may be those of the underlying disease or those of hypotension or hypoxia. The severity of signs varies both with the degree and with the rate of onset of anemia. Acute massive blood loss through hemorrhage may result in rapid death from hypovolemia and hypoxia before any drop in Hb or PCV is evident. In this situation, loss of plasma volume occurs with loss of red cells. Blood flow may be redirected to the brain, heart, and other organs most vulnerable to hypoxemia. The pallor that is noted when one examines the mucous membranes is not caused by thin blood, but rather by reduced perfusion of the superficial vasculature.

If the onset of anemia is slow as with decreased red cell production, clinical signs are minimal until the anemia is severe. Plasma volume may remain normal. Compensatory changes in the respiratory rate, heart rate, cardiac output, and oxygen delivery to tissues protect the patient from some of the signs of anemia. For example, in some species, an increase in 2,3-DPG causes a shift in the oxygen dissociation curve to the right. This allows for easier release of oxygen into the tissues. Tachypnea, tachycardia, and increased cardiac output can compensate to some extent, but eventually decompensate if the anemia is progressive. Anemic patients may show only minimal signs at rest, but show more pronounced signs if stressed or forced to exercise. The behavior of an anemic cat illustrates this point most dramatically: As the red cell number drops over time, the cat will withdraw and sleep more. By the time an owner realizes that a problem exists, the Hct may be <10%. When the cat is taken to the veterinarian, examined, and restrained for blood collection, it can suddenly collapse. One must use caution in working with severely anemic animals, because any medical intervention can increase stress.

Weakness and pale mucous membranes are present with anemia of any cause. A systolic heart murmur related to abnormal closure of the heart valves from low blood viscosity may be heard. In chronic anemia, cardiac hypertrophy results and eventually a "high-output" circulatory failure occurs. The retinal vessels may be less prominent than usual, and occasionally retinal hemorrhages occur. Some anemic animals, especially cats, develop pica. They eat dirt or litter, or lick the floor or walls, perhaps from some instinctive search for nutrients. The reason for this is not known; it does not correlate with any known deficiency in the diet. Iron supplementation does not resolve the clinical signs.

Evaluation of the Anemic Patient

When presented with an animal with weakness and pale mucous membranes, one must first determine whether the cause is anemia or decreased tissue perfusion from shock, hypotension or hypovolemia. The PCV and TP concentration usually will differentiate these conditions. The exception is the animal with acute blood loss. If the bleeding is external, the diagnosis is usually obvious; if it is into a body cavity or the gastrointestinal tract, additional tests will be needed to confirm this. If the patient is found to be anemic and the cause is not known, the most important first step is to decide whether the anemia is regenerative or whether it is nonregenerative (**Part C**). The blood smear from a patient with regenerative anemia may show anisocytosis, polychromasia and macrocytosis, suggesting that reticulocytosis is present. The reticulocyte count is the best indicator of regeneration.

If no sign of internal or external blood loss is found in an animal with reticulocytosis, hemolytic anemia is likely. The term *hemolysis* encompasses all mechanisms that cause red cells to die prematurely. Destruction may be caused by an abnormality within the red cell itself or by external factors acting on the red cell. Hemolysis from any cause may be associated with icterus (jaundice) which occurs when large numbers of red cells are destroyed rapidly, but icterus may also occur with hepatic disease or biliary tract obstruction. Additional laboratory tests are required to evaluate these possibilities.

If the anemia is nonregenerative, the bone marrow is not making enough red cells, either because of a lack of erythropoietin stimulation or because of a failure to respond to erythropoietin from causes such as primary marrow failure, hematopoietic malignancy, or toxic or infectious marrow suppression. Treatment and prognosis vary with the cause of anemia, so an accurate diagnosis is critically important.

Acute Blood Loss

Acute Blood Loss

Prior to blood loss:

Assume blood volume 7% body weight
HCT 40%
Hb 13.3gm/dL
RBC count 5.7 x 10^6/μL
Total protein concentration 7gm/dL
 (Loss of 50% blood volume)

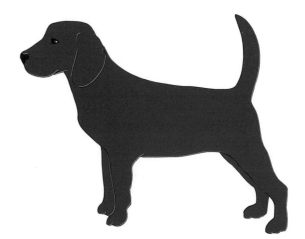

Immediately after blood loss:

Blood volume 3.5% body weight
HCT 40%
Hb 13.3gm/dL
RBC count 5.7 x 10^6/μL
Total protein concentration 7gm/dL
Increased heart rate
Decreased blood pressure

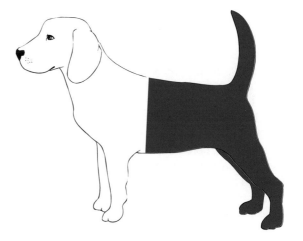

24 hours after blood loss:

Assume fluid intake continues.
(Numbers below approximate depending
on fluid intake of replacement)

Assume blood volume 7% body weight
HCT 20%
Hb 6.7gm/dL
RBC count 2.8 x 10^6/μL
Total protein concentration 4gm/dL

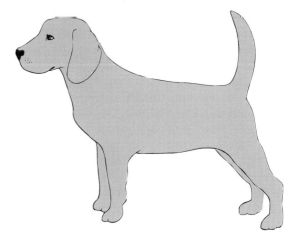

Blood loss may be acute or chronic, each with differing signs and laboratory findings. Trauma and hemorrhage during surgery are common causes. A diagnosis of acute blood loss is obvious after a major vessel is severed in a traumatic incident. Internal blood loss, such as hemorrhage into the abdominal cavity from a ruptured spleen, or bleeding into the stomach or intestinal lumen from an ulcer or tumor, can be more difficult to detect. Another cause of blood loss is a coagulopathy such as decreased platelets (thrombocytopenia) or clotting factors. A clue that a coagulopathy might be present would be if hemorrhage occurs from more than 1 site. Additional coagulation tests can confirm a diagnosis of coagulopathy (see Chapters 42 and 43).

Response to Acute Blood Loss

Normal animals can withstand the loss of 25%–30% of their total blood volume without replacement with blood or intravenous fluid. Animals have more than twice the number of red cells necessary for tissue oxygenation, so the biggest concern with acute blood loss is decreased circulatory volume, blood pressure, and tissue perfusion. Some species such as the dog and the horse have large stores of red cells in the spleen. Epinephrine release at the time of hemorrhage causes contraction of the spleen and release of these cells into the circulation within minutes. Epinephrine may also cause physiological leukocytosis with neutrophilia and perhaps lymphocytosis. Thrombocytosis may occur because of a large, readily available reserve supply in the spleen. In addition, epinephrine increases blood pressure and heart and respiratory rates and causes peripheral vasoconstriction to divert blood flow to the vital organs.

Acute hemorrhage is associated with normal red cell number, size, Hb, and morphology. An animal could bleed to death with no drop in the Hct, Hb, or RBC count, because plasma is lost in the same proportion as red cells (**Figure**). Measuring the Hct or total protein concentration is of no value in monitoring the severity of blood loss in an acutely bleeding animal. The best objective indicator of the severity of acute blood loss is blood pressure measurement.

After hemorrhage into the thoracic or abdominal cavity, the blood initially clots and then is defibrinated, returning to a liquid state and leaving most of the red cells intact. The plasma and about 50% of the red blood cells will re-enter the circulation after several hours. If blood loss occurs into tissues rather than into a body cavity, red cells are not able to reenter the circulation. Destruction of red cells results in bruising after hemorrhage into the skin or subcutaneous tissue.

Within a few hours after blood loss, as fluid shifts occur, the Hct begins to drop. Assuming that fluid intake is continued, the drop occurs gradually over 2–3 days. Concentrations of albumin and other serum proteins decrease as well, but up to 50% of the lost albumin shifts from the interstitium as osmotic equilibrium is re-established. Increased synthesis of albumin begins in approximately 48 hours. Erythropoietin levels begin to rise within about 6 hours, but 3–4 days are required for increased numbers of reticulocytes to enter the circulation. As the reticulocyte count begins to rise, the anemia becomes macrocytic (increased MCV) and normochromic or hypochromic, and the Hct returns to normal in 1–2 weeks.

Enough residual storage iron is present in normal animals to respond to a single episode of acute blood loss. Supplementation with iron is not necessary unless hemorrhage persists or recurs.

Hemorrhagic Shock

The clinical manifestation of hemorrhagic shock may become evident when >30% of the blood volume is lost acutely, especially if the animal must exercise or is emotionally stressed. Initial signs of acute blood loss anemia are tachycardia, tachypnea, weak pulses, pale mucous membranes, and hypotension. Compensatory changes are increased cardiac output and increased oxygen extraction in the tissues. Renal blood flow is maintained initially by reflex relaxation of the afferent arterioles, but if blood pressure drops significantly, urine production decreases to maintain circulatory volume. Most of the circulation is diverted to maintain perfusion of the brain and heart. If hemorrhagic shock is untreated, vasomotor failure ensues, followed by acidosis and the formation of disseminated microthrombi from slowed blood flow and release of various cytokines from hypoxic tissues. Capillary permeability increases, and damaged endothelial cells begin to leak fluid into the tissues. In the lungs, this accumulation of fluid and protein in the interstitial spaces results in dyspnea and further hypoxia, a condition called *adult respiratory distress syndrome* (ARDS). Hypoxic damage to the intestinal mucosa allows leakage of fluid into the lumen as well as invasion of bacteria and endotoxin into the circulation. The significance of the loss of the normal osmotic gradient between plasma and interstitium is that blood volume no longer can be restored effectively. This catastrophic syndrome is known as *irreversible shock*.

Treatment

The goal of treatment is to stop the bleeding and to restore blood volume and oxygen delivery to the tissues. This can be accomplished initially by administering crystalloid fluids such as normal saline solution, or colloids such as dextrans or hetastarch. Dogs are known to survive a 50% loss of blood volume, and baboons have survived removal of blood to a Hct of 15%, if blood volume was maintained with colloids. It is likely that transfusion with red blood cells would be required if blood loss exceeds 50% of the total blood volume.

Plasma transfusion is needed only in the presence of massive bleeding. Coagulation factors comprise the limiting factor, but a normal animal will not become depleted until two-thirds of the clotting factors are lost. Treatment must be administered as soon as possible after hemorrhage occurs, before the normal compensatory mechanisms are overwhelmed.

Ch11 Iron Metabolism

The Iron Cycle

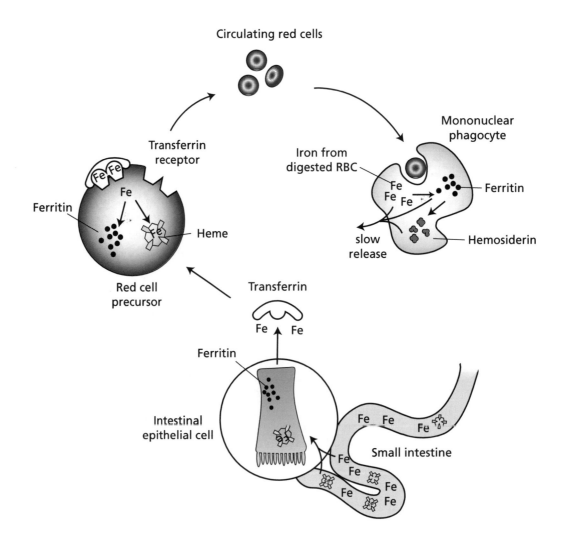

Iron is by far the most abundant heavy metal in the body, and is necessary for the production of hemoglobin. Without it, red cells would not be able to carry and deliver oxygen. Iron is admitted to the body through a complex mechanism of checkpoints that serve also to protect against the toxicity of free ferric ions. The heme molecule has iron in the center, surrounded by 4 pyrrole groups. About 1 mg of iron is needed for every milliliter of red cells produced. Almost all of this iron is obtained by efficient recycling from old red cells.

No mechanism exists for excretion of iron, although small amounts are lost daily from desquamation of intestinal and skin epithelial cells, and additional iron may be lost through bleeding. Carnivores typically ingest more iron than herbivores, but the amount of iron absorbed through the gastrointestinal tract is carefully regulated by need, to avoid iron overload. Studies have shown that while normal dogs absorb little iron, the rate of absorption increases 5–15-fold when iron deficiency is present. In most species, 5%–10% of available dietary iron is absorbed. The exact mechanism for this controlled absorption is not totally clear, but probably depends on the concentration of cytoplasmic iron in the intestinal mucosal cells. Iron is incorporated into the villus cells as these cells are formed in the crypts of Lieberkühn (**Figure**). The iron is picked up as needed as the intestinal cells mature and progress up the crypts. Cytoplasmic iron is primarily in the form of ferritin, an accessible storage form containing multiple molecules of iron in a protein shell.

Most iron absorption takes place in the duodenum and upper jejunum. The normal acid pH of the stomach stabilizes iron complexes in the food and improves absorption. Meat is an excellent source of iron in that heme is absorbed intact. From vegetable sources, iron is absorbed in the ferrous form and then is oxidized to the ferric form. Absorption may be increased by reducing substances such as ascorbate. Absorption may be decreased in an alkaline environment as when antacid therapy is used frequently over a long period of time. In this case, the iron is transformed to an insoluble form that is not absorbed. Iron homeostasis is dependent on 2 iron-sequestering proteins, transferrin and ferritin. Ferritin with its outer protein coat, apoferritin, is responsible for safeguarding iron entry into the body and for keeping the surplus in an accessible storage form. Transferrin transports and recycles iron between plasma and cells. The rates of production of both ferritin and transferrin are regulated by iron concentrations.

All absorbed free iron is bound to transferrin, a β-globulin, and transported to sites in macrophages of the marrow, and to a lesser extent, in the liver and spleen where it is stored as ferritin. Ferritin is visible only by electron microscopy, but circulating ferritin can be measured in the serum. If in the 3–4-day life span of the mucosal cell the iron is not absorbed, the unused ferritin is sloughed into the intestinal lumen and lost.

The transferrin releases the iron and is recycled to scavenge for free iron. Transferrin is produced in the liver in inverse proportion to hepatic iron content; more transferrin is produced in states of low iron, and normally about one-third of transferrin is saturated with iron. Transferrin is a true transport protein. It is not destroyed in the process but is recycled to pick up more iron. The normal concentration of iron in the plasma is about 100 μg/dL.

Developing red cells possess transferrin receptors, the density of the receptors being proportional to the amount of hemoglobin being synthesized at that time. Transferrin attaches to the receptors, enters the cell through invaginations in the cell membrane, releases its iron, and leaves. As red cells become mature, these receptors are lost.

Once the need for marrow iron is filled, saturated transferrin will deposit iron as ferritin in macrophages in the liver and spleen or in hepatic parenchymal cells. During storage, ferritin molecules can become packed within lysosomes to become larger aggregates called *hemosiderin*, which is visible by light microscopy as golden granules on hematoxylin and eosin–stained slides or as blue material when stained with Prussian blue. About 90% of the iron used for new red cell production comes from old red cells. When senescent red cells are removed from the circulation by macrophages in the spleen, heme separates from globin, the heme ring opens, and iron is released into the cytoplasm of the macrophage. Most of the iron is then picked up by transferrin and carried back to the marrow to start the cycle again. Most of the iron present at birth remains for the life of the individual. The iron cycle is so efficient that, in humans, only about 1 mg of iron must be absorbed from the intestine daily to replace losses.

In young animals, very little storage iron is present, and milk is a poor source of iron. In rapidly growing animals, the rate of growth may exceed the availability of iron. Young animals are more likely than adults to become iron deficient whenever blood is lost. Absorption of iron from the intestine in young animals is much greater than that in adults. Excessive supplementation of the diet can cause the immature intestine to absorb too much and result in iron toxicity. Excessive absorption of iron rarely occurs in the normal adult, and iron overload only occurs in situations where injectable iron supplements are used or multiple red cell transfusions are given. Iron stored in excess of that needed is irritating and eventually results in cirrhosis of the liver.

Hereditary hemochromatosis is a disorder primarily of humans in which excess iron is absorbed by the intestine regardless of need. A similar syndrome has been reported in mynah birds, and rarely in Salers cattle and horses. Excessive iron, over time, damages primarily the liver and the heart. Human patients also have developed a bronze skin color from iron deposition (bronze diabetes), and some eventually died of malignant hepatomas.

Sequence of Events in Iron Deficiency Caused by Slow Bleeding from Gastrointestinal Tract

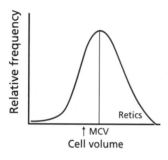

Positive test for blood in stool
Reticulocytosis,↑ RDW
↑ MCV, polychromasia, normal Hct
Thrombocytosis

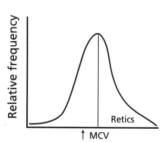

Depletion of storage iron in marrow
Decreased serum ferritin
↓ TP
Rest same as above

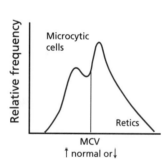

Decreased serum iron, ↓ saturation of transferrin
Some microcytic cells,↑ RDW
MCV ↑, or normal
Rest same as above

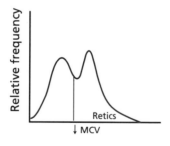

Anemia
↓ MCV, ↓MCHC (microcytic hypochromic)
Rest sames as above

Whenever the need for iron to make new red cells exceeds the availability, iron is first mobilized from storage sites (**Figure**). Initially, the Hct and red cell indices remain normal, but serum ferritin concentration and the amount of stainable iron (with Prussian blue stain) in the marrow begin to decrease. Normal cats have very little storage iron in the marrow, so evaluation of iron stores is not easily performed in cats. In the marrow, as the deficiency becomes more severe, decreased hemoglobin synthesis leads to a retention of a viable nucleus beyond the normal number of cell divisions. The developing red cell continues to divide, "hoping" to increase the concentration of hemoglobin in each red cell. The additional divisions result in smaller than normal red cells (microcytosis), and with a decreased concentration of hemoglobin per cell (MCHC) resulting in hypochromasia. If the decrease in iron is due to chronic blood loss, oral intake of iron tends to continue and reticulocytosis persists. If significant reticulocytosis is present, the large size (macrocytosis) of the reticulocytes can mask the presence of microcytosis if only the MCV is measured. Examination of the red cell histogram may show several peaks, with large reticulocytes, normal red cells, and microcytic cells, with an increased RDW. Initially, compensatory mechanisms allow the iron-deficient animal to maintain a normal Hct despite all of the morphological and structural changes that are occurring. The poorly structured red cells have a tendency to fragment in the circulation, resulting in the appearance of schistocytes and an overall description of poikilocytosis. When the marrow can no longer keep up with losses, serum iron concentration decreases, and the Hct drops. The production of transferrin increases in the liver so that more iron can be absorbed by the intestine and transported to the marrow. If the iron deficiency is caused by decreased intake, reticulocytosis may not occur.

Nutritional Deficiency of Iron

Baby pigs are especially prone to iron deficiency, because of their rapid growth rate and because sow's milk is very low in iron. In the past when pigs were raised in farmyards, iron deficiency was not a problem because baby pigs root in the soil, and the sow's belly is often covered with dirt, which contains a high concentration of iron. If baby pigs are raised on clean concrete floors without access to soil, essentially all will become anemic, and some will die if iron supplements are not provided. This is an example of modern "improvements" causing a new problem. Nutritional iron deficiency is less common in other species, although a small drop in Hct is common in nursing animals. The Hct self-corrects at the time of weaning. In humans, nutritional iron deficiency can occur with some unusual vegetarian diets, especially in rapidly growing children and menstruating women.

Chronic Blood Loss

Iron deficiency occurs most commonly as a result of chronic blood loss, especially through the gastrointestinal tract. In young animals, blood-sucking intestinal parasites such as hookworms in dogs and stomach worms in ruminants are the most likely reasons for gastrointestinal blood loss. A single hookworm may remove up to 0.8 mL of blood per day. External parasites such as fleas and lice may be so numerous as to cause significant blood loss. In older animals, ulcerated tumors, especially leiomyomas, leiomyosarcomas, and adenocarcinomas of the stomach or intestines, are the most common reasons for gastrointestinal bleeding. Ulcers occur occasionally as a primary problem, but less commonly than in humans.

Internal bleeding as might occur into a body cavity will not result in iron deficiency since iron is reabsorbed. Chronic hemoglobinuria will deplete iron but usually not to the point of causing iron deficiency.

Iatrogenic blood loss anemia can occur occasionally when multiple blood samples are drawn for laboratory testing of hospitalized small dogs or cats. For example, 10 mL of blood drawn daily for 4 days from a cat weighing 6 lb represents about 20% of the total blood volume.

Laboratory Findings

Iron deficiency is the most common cause of microcytic hypochromic anemia, although it has been found in patients with copper deficiency or hepatic portosystemic vascular anomalies. Microcytic red cells are normal in the Akita and Sheba breeds of dogs, so indices must be interpreted with caution in these breeds.

Typical laboratory findings include anemia and decreased serum iron levels, decreased stainable iron in the bone marrow, and decreased serum ferritin levels. The serum iron is equal to the amount of iron that is bound to transferrin. In some species the total iron-binding capacity (TIBC), equal to the amount of iron that potentially could be bound to transferrin if the transferrin were 100% saturated with iron, is a useful measure. The percent saturation (percent saturation = serum iron/TIBC) as an indicator of iron deficiency is useful in some species. In dogs, iron deficiency is associated with a decreased percent saturation of transferrin and normal TIBC. Most other species show a decreased percent saturation and increased TIBC.

If iron deficiency is caused by chronic blood loss, thrombocytosis commonly occurs. This is probably a reactive increase secondary to chronic low-grade consumption of platelets at the bleeding site and increased production in the marrow. Another rather consistent finding with chronic blood loss is hypoproteinemia since plasma protein is lost along with red cells. Edema may develop in animals with severe hypoproteinemia. This has been observed primarily in ruminants.

Treatment of iron deficiency must address the cause. Cure will not be obtained unless the cause of blood loss is removed. Iron supplementation sometimes has been recommended empirically for patients anemic from any cause. Additional iron is not useful to the patient and may cause gastric irritation or iron overload.

Ch13 Hemolytic Anemia

A   Intravascular Hemolysis

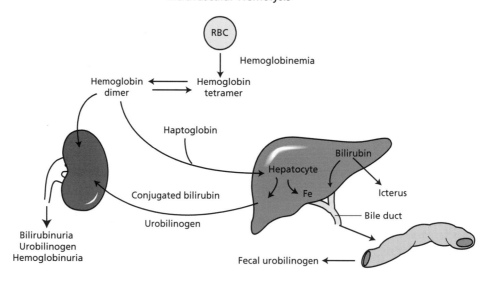

Extravascular Hemolysis

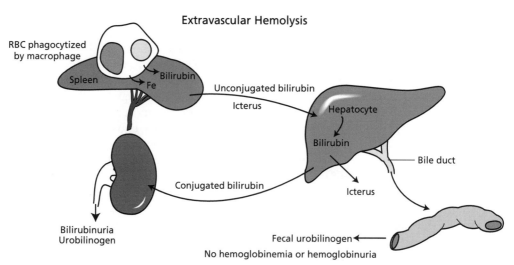

B   Signs of Hemolysis on the Hemogram

1. Signs of regenerative anemia

   Macrocytosis
   Increased MCV
   Reticulocytosis
   Anisocytosis
   Leukocytosis
   Thrombocytosis
   Polychromasia
   Decreased myeloid/erythroid (M/E) ratio in
     marrow because of erythroid hyperplasia

2. More specific signs of hemolysis

   Hyperbilirubinemia
   Increased urinary urobilinogen
   Icterus
   Spherocytosis
   Hemoglobinemia
   Hemoglobinuria

Hemolytic anemia is associated with premature death or accelerated destruction of red cells and may be caused by a defect in the red cell itself (intrinsic) or by external factors acting on the red cell (extrinsic). Many of the intrinsic disorders are hereditary metabolic conditions such as porphyria, in which the hemoglobin itself is abnormal, and pyruvate kinase or phosphofructokinase deficiency, in which red cell metabolism is abnormal. In these conditions, the cells cannot derive full benefit from glucose metabolism, and ATP production is decreased. The cells do not survive as long as normal red cells, and if cells are not produced by the marrow at the same rate that they are destroyed, anemia results. Extrinsic causes of hemolysis occur more frequently than do intrinsic disorders. With extrinsic disorders, the normal red cells are destroyed by antibodies, toxins, or other factors. If a compatible red blood cell transfusion is given to a patient with an intrinsic disorder, the transfused cells would have a normal survival time, whereas the survival time would be shortened in a patient with an extrinsic disorder.

The mechanism of hemolysis is similar to the destruction of senescent red cells in the normal animal. The spleen is the major site of removal of senescent or defective red cells. Certain alterations in red cells predispose them to destruction. These include coating of the cell by antibody, decreased surface area–volume ratio, altered membrane structure, and oxidant stress. A decreased surface area–volume ratio occurs when part of the cell membrane is lost. This can happen in immune-mediated hemolytic anemia when the surface of the red cell is coated by antibodies. When splenic macrophages attach, some red cells escape before being phagocytized, but part of the cell membrane may be left behind. The membrane can repair the defect, leaving a smaller, more spherical cell called a *spherocyte*. This same effect can be seen with exposure of senescent antigens and spherocyte formation. The spherocyte is less deformable and more likely to be removed during subsequent passages through the splenic sinusoids. A decreased surface area–volume ratio can also occur when the volume of the red cell is increased. This can occur with water intoxication from excessive oral intake or from administration of hypotonic intravenous fluids, or in freshwater drowning. Excessive and rapid influx of hypotonic fluid or water causes increased uptake into the red cells and eventual rupture.

An altered membrane structure with decreased elasticity of the membrane proteins can occur in aged red cells with decreased ATP. Normally ATP maintains flexibility of the cell membranes. When this is lost, red cells are easily trapped and removed. In patients with liver disease, increased viscosity of the membrane lipids causes cells to become rigid and prone to removal. Membrane integrity may be damaged by toxins, infections, parasites, or trauma. A hemolytic toxin is produced by *Clostridium hemolyticum*, the cause of bacillary hemoglobinuria in cattle. Mothballs containing naphthalene have caused hemolysis in dogs. Examples of infections causing hemolysis are equine infectious anemia and leptospirosis. Red cell parasites such as babesiosis, malaria, and hemobartonellosis cause hemolytic anemia. Direct trauma to red cells occurs when abnormal endothelium (microangiopathic hemolysis) or fibrin clots are encountered. Examples include hemangiosarcoma and disseminated intravascular coagulopathy.

Oxidant stress on red blood cells occurs when heme iron is oxidized to the ferric (3+) form, known as methemoglobin, instead of the reduced form (2+) needed to carry oxygen. Sometimes the methemoglobin becomes denatured and forms precipitates called *Heinz bodies,* colorless inclusions protruding from the red cell membrane.

Hemolytic anemias may be divided into 2 types depending on the major site of destruction of red cells (**Part A**). If red cells are lysed within the vasculature, the result is *intravascular* hemolysis. If red cells are trapped and removed by splenic macrophages before lysis, the hemolysis is termed *extravascular*. This distinction is important in determining the cause of the anemia since one or the other type is usually characteristic of specific etiologies. It may also be prognostic since intravascular hemolysis tends to be more severe.

In intravascular hemolysis, free hemoglobin binds to heptoglobin for transport to the liver, but only a limited amount of heptoglobin is present. Excessive free hemoglobin dissociates into αβ dimers, which are small enough to pass through the glomerular filtrate into the urine. Characteristic findings of intravascular hemolysis are red plasma (hemoglobinemia) and urine (hemoglobinuria) because of the presence of free hemoglobin. Sometimes the observation of hemoglobinuria might be the first indication that hemolysis is occurring. One must differentiate hemoglobinuria from hematuria (blood in the urine). If the urine sample with hematuria is centrifuged, intact red cells settle to the bottom whereas with hemoglobinuria, the hemoglobin remains in solution. In both cases, a urine test for blood would be positive.

In most hemolytic processes, the red cells are trapped and removed by macrophages in the sinuses of the spleen, and to a lesser extent in the liver (extravascular hemolysis). With extravascular hemolysis, hemoglobinemia and hemoglobinuria are not present. Splenomegaly is more likely to occur with extravascular hemolysis but could be present in either type. Icterus may be present with hemolysis of any cause. Other changes in red cell morphology might be seen and indicate specific causes of hemolytic anemia described in later chapters (**Part B**).

In a normal individual the bone marrow can increase its output of red cells by about 6–8 times the normal rate. Thus, the red cell life span could be reduced to one-eighth normal before a drop in the PCV occurs. Examination of the bone marrow is usually not of value in evaluating the cause of any regenerative anemia since one would just see signs of increased erythroid production. For most hemolytic anemias, the history, physical examination, and evaluation of the hemogram and especially the blood smear will provide clues to the cause.

Ch14   Immune-mediated Hemolysis

The Coomb's (Antiglobulin) Test

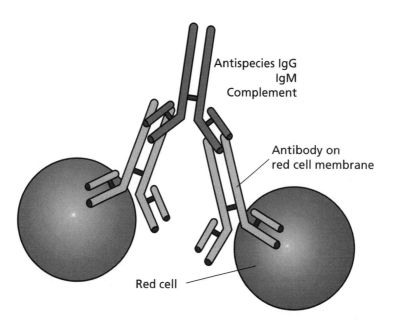

Antispecies IgG
IgM
Complement

Antibody on
red cell membrane

Red cell

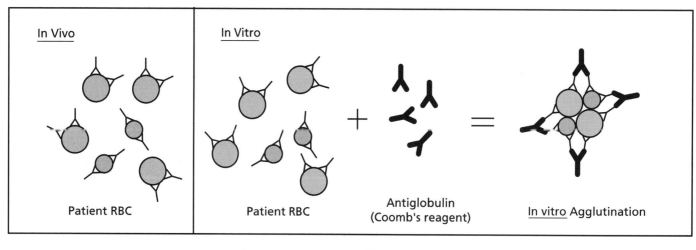

In Vivo

Patient RBC

In Vitro

Patient RBC   +   Antiglobulin
(Coomb's reagent)   =   In vitro Agglutination

Legend: $\curlywedge$ = IgG $\mathbf{\curlywedge}$ = anti- IgG   ◯ = mature RBC   ⬤ = spherocyte

Immunologic destruction of red cells, usually called *autoimmune* (AIHA) or *immune-mediated hemolytic anemia* (IMHA), is probably the most common cause of hemolytic anemia in the dog. It also occurs in humans, cats, and horses. Normal clearance of aged red cells is mediated by antibody directed against senescent red cell antigens, which allows these cells to be recognized by the mononuclear phagocytic system. The senescent antigen is most likely a membrane protein that becomes expressed as the cell ages.

IMHA associated with complement-fixing IgG or IgM can cause intravascular hemolysis, sometimes associated with autoagglutination of red cells that may be visible grossly or microscopically. Intravascular hemolysis results in the formation of vasoactive and chemotactic substances that can be harmful. Most dogs with IMHA have extravascular hemolysis, in which phagocytic cells in the spleen or liver remove red cells coated with antibody. The spleen is the primary site of removal of cells that are coated with IgG, are abnormally shaped, or have decreased deformability. Spherocytes are small dense rigid red cells that are formed when macrophages remove part of the membrane. Spherocytes become trapped in small vascular spaces in the spleen, where they can be phagocytized along with normal red cells that can be trapped secondarily. With increasing numbers of IgG molecules bound to the cell, more complement activation occurs and the survival of sensitized red cells is progressively shortened.

Causes

The causes of IMHA are not understood but may be associated with other autoimmune disorders, or secondary to other diseases, viral infections, drugs, or toxins. Imbalances between suppressor and helper T-cell function have been suspected. Impaired suppressor T-cell function has been demonstrated in certain strains of mice and in some human patients, suggesting that some individuals may be genetically predisposed to develop IMHA. The antigens toward which the antibodies are directed are usually not specific to the patient, but shared by others. It is unlikely that a change in red cell membrane by an exogenous cause triggers IMHA, since normal red cells transfused into patients with IMHA usually are destroyed, as well as their own cells. It is more likely that these agents share antigenic determinants with red cell membrane proteins and cause a cross-reacting antibody response that destroys the red cells. The passive adherence of immune complexes or drugs to the red cell also can predispose to hemolysis. Antibodies involved in canine IMHA are primarily complement-fixing IgG. Some association has been made between recent vaccination with modified live-virus vaccines and the development of IMHA in dogs. Some reports also have mentioned an increased prevalence of IMHA after parvovirus was added to standard vaccines.

Clinical and Laboratory Findings

Either sex can be affected, but most of the cases are in middle-aged females. A higher incidence has been reported in cocker spaniels and poodles. Signs such as weakness, lethargy, and anorexia are vague, but if hemolysis is acute and severe, fever, hemoglobinuria, icterus, or vomiting can occur. Splenomegaly may be present.

Typical laboratory findings are macrocytic, hypochromic, or normochromic anemia; reticulocytosis; spherocytosis; anisocytosis; and polychromasia. Massive hemolysis, especially intravascular, can cause a severe leukocytosis with neutrophilia and a left shift and a febrile response that might be confused with an infection. Circulating nucleated red cells may be present but are not an indicator of a regenerative anemia. Significant anisocytosis and increased RDW occur because of the presence of large reticulocytes and small spherocytes. However, the MCV is increased or normal, not decreased. The finding of spherocytosis strongly supports a diagnosis of IMHA. The MCHC may be decreased if significant reticulocytosis is present, or artifactually increased if hemoglobinemia is present. Spontaneous clumping or autoagglutination of red cells may occur when blood is placed in an EDTA tube or on a slide. This can be caused by either antibody (usually IgG plus complement) or increased rouleau formation usually secondary to elevated serum protein levels. Rouleaux tend to disperse when the blood is diluted in 3–4 volumes of saline, whereas true antibody-mediated agglutination remains. The presence of autoagglutination in a dog with signs of hemolytic anemia can be considered diagnostic of IMHA. Thrombocytopenia, thromboembolism, and disseminated intravascular coagulopathy (DIC) have been recognized as complications of IMHA. Thrombocytopenia can be immune mediated or from consumption of platelets by DIC.

Most dogs with IMHA will have positive direct antiglobulin text (DAT), sometimes called a *Coombs' test* (**Figure**). No correlation seems to exist between the strength of the reaction and the severity of clinical disease. The reagent must be species specific. Most standard canine reagents are pooled antisera directed against canine IgG, IgM, and complement so that cells with either immunoglobulin or complement will be positive. The DAT result may be negative in some anemias clinically compatible with IMHA. Some reasons for real or apparent "false-negative" reactions are incorrect diagnosis, too few antibody molecules to detect, spontaneous elution of the antibody from the red cell, or laboratory procedural errors.

Clinically significant antibodies are active at 37°C, the temperature at which the test is routinely run. In contrast, many normal dogs have antibodies that cause spontaneous agglutination of their own red cells or those of other dogs at 4°C. Cold hemagglutinin disease and IMHA associated with cold-reacting antibodies is rarely seen in dogs. Hemolysis occurs at cold temperatures, and plugging of capillaries in cold parts of the body causes necrosis of the tips of the ears, tail, and toes.

Not all dogs with IMHA will have reticulocytosis. If reticulocytes are destroyed in the marrow, the anemia will appear nonregenerative (*see* Chapter 20).

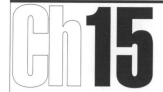

Blood Group Antigens and Transfusions

Genesis of Transfusion Reactions

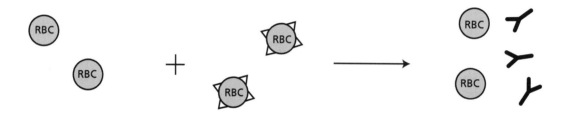

Type-A negative dog

Transfusion with A-positve RBCs
No reaction.

Development of anti-A antibodies

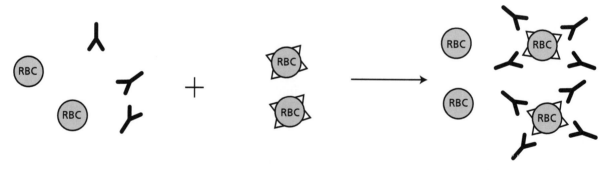

Type-A negative dog or
Type-B cat with anti-A antibodies

Repeat A-positive transfusion (dog)
or first type-A transfusion (cat)

Binding of antibody and clinical
hemolytic transfusion reaction

Immune-mediated hemolysis frequently is associated with the presence of autoantibodies, antibodies produced by a patient, to an antigen present on his or her own red cells. Alloimmune hemolysis occurs if an antibody produced by one individual causes hemolysis of red cells in another individual. The primary causes of alloimmune hemolysis are hemolytic transfusion reactions and hemolytic disease of the newborn.

The earliest recorded transfusions were composed of milk or wine, and later by transfusion of animal blood into humans. Because problems were encountered and no benefit was observed, research then moved to transfusion from a donor of the same species as the recipient. Initially blood was taken and immediately given to the recipient because of a lack of knowledge of anticoagulants and the mechanisms for storage. Despite dramatic improvement observed in some cases, occasionally the recipient suffered from acute, sometimes fatal hemolytic transfusion reactions. Not until Landsteiner discovered human ABO blood group antigens early in the 20th century were these reactions explained and in most cases, prevented.

Blood group variability exists in humans as well as domestic animals, including birds. Although they are designated by letters of the alphabet, the antigens differ between species even if they are named by the same letter. The surface of the red cell membrane contains many different components that may or may not be present on the surface of red cells of other members of the same species. Some of these components are antigenic when injected into the recipient of a blood transfusion. Blood group antigens are polysaccharides, with the genetically controlled terminal sugar defining the specificity. Antigens identical to the human A and B antigens are widespread on the surface of some bacteria or plants so that babies encounter these soon after birth and produce antibodies to the antigens that they lack. Most of these antigens are inherited independently so that any individual will have some antigens and lack others. Some antigens may have >1 allele at a specific locus. One allele may be dominant over another so that a heterozygous individual would have the same phenotype (blood type) as would another individual homozygous for the dominant allele. In other cases, alleles may be codominant. These differences are illustrated by the AB system in humans and cats. In humans, A and B are codominant, whereas in the cat, A is dominant to B and the AB allele is separate and recessive to A but dominant to B. Group O red cells of humans lack both A and B antigens. Nothing comparable to O has been identified in cats. So far the cat is known to possess only the AB system, while humans and most other species studied have many more. In humans, the prevalence of certain blood group antigens varies between nationalities. In cats, the prevalence of the B antigen is very low (<1%) in domestic shorthair and longhair breeds, whereas it ranges as high as 25%–50% in some breeds such as British shorthair, Abyssinian, Persian, Himalayan, and Devon Rex.

For both human and cat A and B antigens, naturally occurring antibodies are present if the antigen is not present. For canine red cell antigens, for non-ABO antigens in humans, and for most red cell antigens of other species, naturally occurring antibodies are not present unless the patient has been sensitized by transfusion or (in some species) by pregnancy. Blood groups of cattle are perhaps the most complex, with >200 phenotypes recognized, involving multiple genes and alleles. The diversity of groups has been utilized as a means of identifying breeds and even individual animals.

For the purposes of transfusion, certain blood group antigens are known to be more "antigenic" (capable of inducing an antibody response) in animals lacking that antigen. An example is DEA (dog erythrocyte antigen) 1.1 (**Figure**). If a dog lacking this antigen is given a transfusion of red cells containing DEA 1.1, it is likely that antibodies will be formed. If this dog receives a later transfusion of DEA 1.1–positive cells after antibodies are formed, an acute hemolytic reaction is likely to occur. In addition to DEA 1.1, 12–14 other red cell antigens have been identified in dogs (and are called DEA followed by a number). These seem to be less capable of inducing an antibody response when transfused into a dog lacking the antigens, but a potential risk does exist for sensitization by any foreign antigen.

Some of the canine red cell antigens are rare (in <5% of dogs) and others are very common (in >98% of dogs). For these antigens, the chances are good that the donor and recipient will match. Other antigens like DEA 1.1 and DEA 7 are present in approximately 40% of the population; so chances of mismatch are higher. If this occurs, antibodies may develop and cause a hemolytic reaction if that antigen is given in a subsequent transfusion. A dog may develop significant antibodies within 7–10 days after such a transfusion. Because it is impossible or impractical to type humans or dogs for all known antigens, potential recipients can be checked for antibodies by reacting the recipient serum with donor red cells (major crossmatch) and looking for agglutination. The crossmatch will not indicate whether antibodies will be formed after foreign antigens are transfused.

Although transfusions are less frequent in large animals such as horses, certain antigens such as A and Q are most antigenic but many other antigens exist. Some naturally occurring antibodies must exist in horses because donor red blood cells that appear compatible on crossmatch are destroyed within a few days after transfusion. Equine donors should be A and Q negative since it is difficult to type recipients in the event of an emergency.

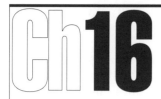

Hemolytic Disease of the Newborn

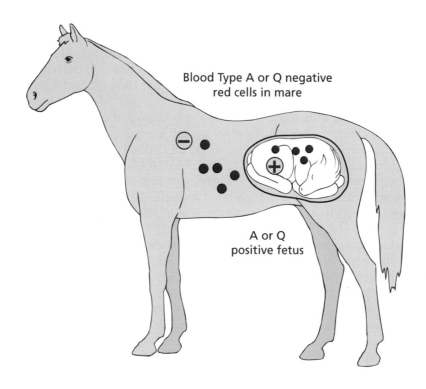

Blood Type A or Q negative
red cells in mare

A or Q
positive fetus

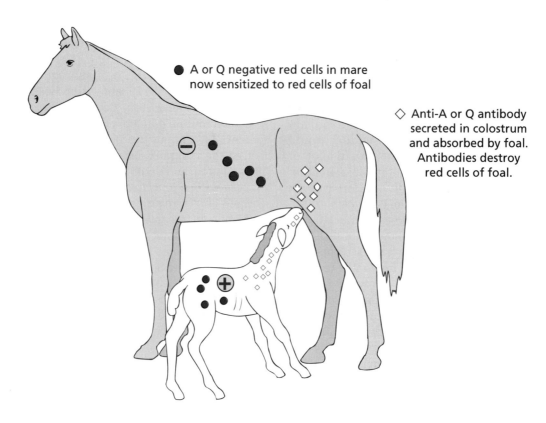

● A or Q negative red cells in mare
now sensitized to red cells of foal

◇ Anti-A or Q antibody
secreted in colostrum
and absorbed by foal.
Antibodies destroy
red cells of foal.

Hemolytic disease of the newborn, also known as neonatal isoerythrolysis (NI), and in humans as erythroblastosis fetalis or Rh disease, is another cause of alloimmune hemolysis. Maternal antibodies form when the mother is sensitized to foreign antigens on the red cells of her fetus. These red cells have been inherited from the sire (**Figure**).

Pathogenesis

Human mothers may become sensitized to certain antigens, most commonly Rh through exposure to fetal red cells during pregnancy or at parturition. Sensitization could also occur from a prior transfusion. If fetal red cells in subsequent pregnancies contain these antigens, maternal antibody may pass through the placenta and cause hemolysis before birth of the fetus. Although Rh is the most common cause of hemolysis in human fetuses, other less-well-known blood group antigens also can cause the same syndrome. Hemolytic disease of the newborn can be caused in the same way in other primates that have the same placental structure as humans.

In other species of animals, the pathogenesis differs in that placental structure does not allow passage of maternal antibodies. Instead, these antibodies are passed in colostrum, and newborn animals can absorb them through the intestine during the first day of life. Gestation is normal and animals are born healthy but develop Coombs-positive hemolytic anemia within hours to days after the first ingestion of colostrum. In horses, this problem has been recognized for >200 years, although the cause was not understood until our knowledge of blood groups developed. The mare is sensitized most commonly by leakage of fetal cells during a prior pregnancy and at parturition, although mares have been known to become sensitized as early as 56 days after conception. First-born foals are seldomly affected. The risk increases with every subsequent pregnancy involving the same sire or one with an identical blood group antigen. The antigens most commonly involved are A, C, and Q. Although hemolytic disease of the newborn can occur in any foal, it is most frequent in thoroughbreds and especially in mules because of greater differences between horse and donkey red cell antigens.

In type B cats, hemolysis can occur in kittens inheriting the A antigen from the sire. The anti-A antibody is present in high titer in all type B cats so prior pregnancy or transfusion is not required for antibodies to form, and hemolysis may occur in the first pregnancy. The anti-B antibody present in Type A cats is not strong enough to cause this problem.

In cattle, use of vaccines (e.g., anaplasmosis) containing blood products has resulted in cows becoming sensitized. If the bull has the same red cell antigens as the vaccine donor, then the calf may share these antigens and develop hemolysis. In dogs, transfusion of DEA 1.1–positive blood can sensitize negative bitches and be a cause of hemolysis should she be bred to a positive male.

In horses, one can detect sensitization of the mare by performing a Coombs' test (*see* Chapter 14) on the sire's red cells mixed with the serum of the mare either before breeding or during pregnancy. If the test result is positive, or if the sire is not available, the red cells of the newborn foal can be tested at birth by reacting them with the serum of the mare. A positive test result indicates that the foal has inherited the sire's antigen and the foal is not allowed to ingest colostrum from the dam. Since the failure to receive colostrum leaves the newborn animal without passive antibody protection from diseases, alternative means of protection must be used. Colostrum negative for antibodies may be stored frozen and used for this purpose or plasma transfusion is given. After the first 48 hours of life, the newborn animal may be allowed to nurse from the dam since antibodies can no longer be absorbed.

In kittens born to a mating of a type B queen and type A tom, typing of the kittens' blood can be done before they are allowed to nurse. Only type B kittens should receive colostrum. Cat breeders are aware of this problem and typically try to breed type B queens to type B males.

Treatment

Affected newborns of any species show evidence of a Coombs-positive intravascular hemolysis developing usually within 12–48 hours after birth. The most vigorous newborn animals may be most severely affected because they take in the greatest quantity of colostrum. Treatment consists of compatible transfusions and supportive care. Saline-washed red cells of the mare are most often used for transfusion. The antibodies are removed with the plasma during washing.

Red Blood Cell Substitutes

Use of Purified Hemoglobin Solution for Transfusion

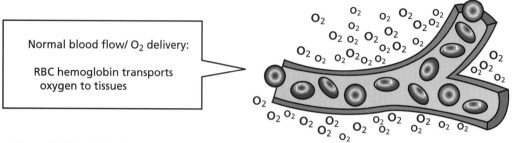

Normal blood flow/ O$_2$ delivery:

RBC hemoglobin transports oxygen to tissues

Hemoglobin within the RBC is responsible for the transport of oxygen from the lungs to the tissue beds via the capillary microcirculation.

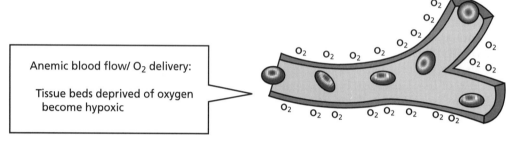

Anemic blood flow/ O$_2$ delivery:

Tissue beds deprived of oxygen become hypoxic

In anemic conditions, oxygen delivery is decreased due to a decrease in circulating RBC's. The microcirculation can partially compensate by directing blood flow to vital tissue beds. Consequently, other tissue beds become deprived of oxygen. The clinical signs of anemia such as pallor, tachycardia, and weakness reflect the decreases in oxygen carrying ability of the blood. In severe cases, anemia can cause organ damage or death.

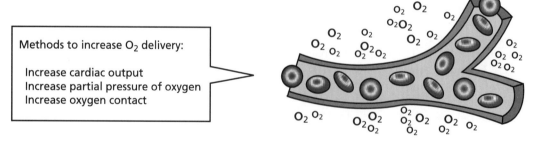

Methods to increase O$_2$ delivery:

Increase cardiac output
Increase partial pressure of oxygen
Increase oxygen contact

Previously, the only way to improve oxygen delivery in anemic animals was to give a blood transfusion, administer crystalloids or colloids to improve blood flow, or increase the partial pressure of oxygen in the blood via delivering an increased fractional inspired concentration of oxygen.

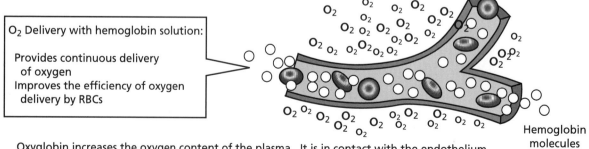

O$_2$ Delivery with hemoglobin solution:

Provides continuous delivery of oxygen
Improves the efficiency of oxygen delivery by RBCs

Hemoglobin molecules

Oxyglobin increases the oxygen content of the plasma. It is in contact with the endothelium of the blood vessels, providing continuous delivery of oxygen to the tissues. By fascilitating diffusion, Oxyglobin improves the efficiency of oxygen delivery by the existing red blood cells.

Because of practical problems associated with finding compatible donors and because of certain diseases known to be transmitted by transfusion, the search for a red cell substitute has been ongoing for >50 years. An ideal substitute would carry and deliver oxygen like red cells, be easy to produce in large quantities, be nonantigenic, and persist in the circulation at least long enough for resuscitation.

Initially hemoglobin solutions were prepared from hemolyzed red cells and infused into experimental animals and human subjects. In addition to its ability to carry oxygen, hemoglobin possesses oncotic properties. Early studies encountered adverse effects such as hypertension, bradycardia, and oliguria, which later were understood to be caused by contamination of the solution with red cell membrane fragments. The early hemoglobin solutions were cleared rapidly by the kidney. Because of these problems, alternative oxygen-carrying substances were sought.

Perfluorocarbons

Similar to Teflon, perfluorocarbons were prepared as emulsions in water. The oxygen in perfluorocarbons is dissolved physically as compared to the chemical binding of oxygen to hemoglobin. Early work in mice given perfluorocarbons looked promising in that the entire blood volume of a mouse could be replaced and the animals could survive if they were kept in an atmosphere of 90%–100% oxygen. However, perfluorocarbons have had limited clinical use because they require very high atmospheric oxygen tension to support delivery of oxygen to tissues of the recipient. They are so inconvenient and impractical that they generally have been discarded except for some use in imaging studies.

Stroma-Free Polymerized Hemoglobin

Interest in hemoglobin solutions as blood substitutes for human use increased greatly after the human immunodeficiency virus was found to be transmissible via transfusion and patients sometimes refused to receive blood. Modifications have been made in hemoglobin solutions to improve safety and efficacy. New filtration techniques are capable of removing the stromal elements that were the likely cause of most of the previously observed adverse effects. Polymerization of hemoglobin dimers allowed the product to persist in the circulation, and the half-life increased from 3–4 hours to approximately 36 hours. An additional problem was encountered with hemoglobin solutions of human origin in that the 2,3-DPG present in normal red cells allowing for release of oxygen in the tissues is missing from purified hemoglobin solutions. For human hemoglobin solutions, an additional step utilizing pyridoxal 5′-phosphate to adhere to 2,3-DPG–binding sites reduced oxygen affinity and allowed oxygen to be released.

One company (Biopure, Cambridge, MA) developed purified, polymerized hemoglobin of bovine origin (Oxyglobin). An advantage of bovine hemoglobin, in addition to its increased availability, is that 2,3-DPG is not required for release of oxygen. Instead, oxygen release is chloride dependent. This product carries and delivers oxygen efficiently and has a 2-year shelf life at room temperatures. Because the structure of the hemoglobin molecule is similar between species, bovine hemoglobin is minimally antigenic when given to humans and domestic animals. This product has been licensed for use in dogs and is currently being tested in cats, horses, birds, and humans. This product is of benefit in veterinary practice because it can be used immediately without need for typing or crossmatching. Its colloidal effects are especially useful in resuscitation after trauma with acute blood loss. In dogs with immune-mediated hemolytic anemia, it may be preferable to transfusions of red cells, which are rapidly hemolyzed.

In the normal animal, hemoglobin within red cells picks up oxygen from the lungs and deposits it in the tissues via the capillary microcirculation (**Figure**). Only a very small amount of oxygen can be carried dissolved in plasma. In the anemic animal, the hemoglobin within each red cell becomes saturated fully with oxygen, but tissue oxygenation is inadequate simply because fewer red cells are present. In hypotension, hypovolemia, or local tissue ischemia, oxygen delivery may be impaired further because of constriction or decreased perfusion of the capillaries. If hemoglobin solution is given, not only does the oxygen content of the plasma improve, but also the delivery of oxygen is easier since the oxygen is already in contact with endothelium and has only to diffuse into the tissues. Because the viscosity of the blood is lower after hemoglobin transfusion than it would be after administration of a comparable volume of blood, perfusion of small capillaries is better.

When hemoglobin solution is given, the patient can be monitored by measuring 1) the Hct to determine the status of the patient's own red cells; 2) the plasma hemoglobin to determine how much of the total hemoglobin is made up of transfused hemoglobin; and 3) the total hemoglobin, which is the best indicator of the patient's overall oxygen-carrying ability. Some serum chemistry values and urine dipstick tests become temporarily invalid after hemoglobin administration. In addition, the MCHC will be increased by the amount of free plasma hemoglobin.

Antibodies to bovine hemoglobin may form, but no clinical manifestations have been observed. Bovine hemoglobin is recommended for one-time use, but experimentally, multiple doses have been given to animals without adverse effects. The purification process is such that known pathogenic organisms do not enter the final product. The question of mad cow disease has been addressed by using closed herds of U.S. origin and carefully controlling the diets of donors. Although hemoglobin solutions can be lifesaving when used as a plasma volume expander in patients with hypovolemic shock, circulatory overload can occur. Patients must be carefully monitored to prevent this problem. Central venous pressure can be monitored and is a sensitive indicator of overdose when large volumes are used.

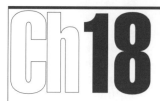

Oxidative Injury to Red Cells

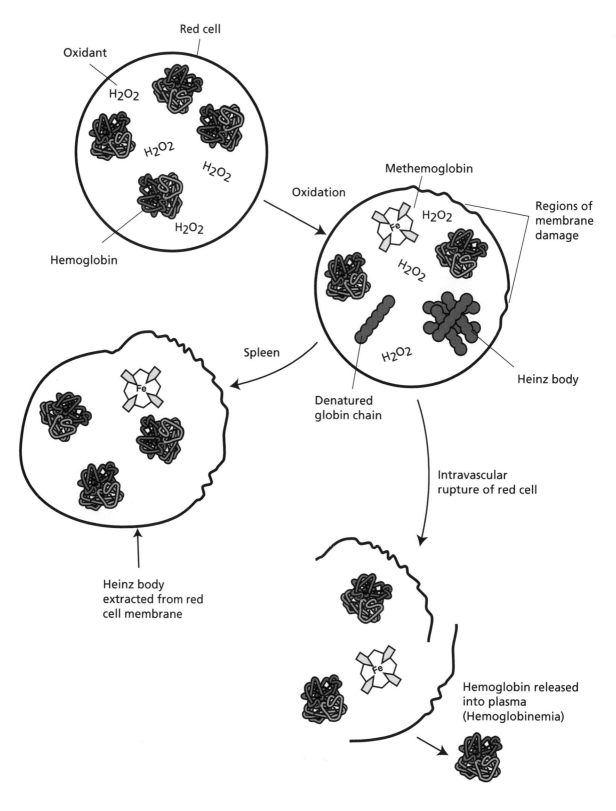

Oxidant Damage of Red Cells

Red cell

Oxidant

H₂O₂

H₂O₂

H₂O₂

H₂O₂

Hemoglobin

Oxidation

Methemoglobin

Fe

H₂O₂

Regions of
membrane
damage

H₂O₂

H₂O₂

Heinz body

Spleen

Denatured
globin chain

Fe

Heinz body
extracted from red
cell membrane

Intravascular
rupture of red cell

Fe

Hemoglobin released
into plasma
(Hemoglobinemia)

Whenever heme iron is oxidized from Fe^{2+} to Fe^{3+}, the hemoglobin is referred to as *methemoglobin* and cannot take up and carry oxygen. This injury occurs within hours after depletion of protective mechanisms such as glutathione within red cells. The process may be reversible if the methemoglobin is reduced back to hemoglobin by the transfer of an electron from NADH to the heme iron atom (see **Figure**). The methemoglobin reductase pathway provides much of the necessary reducing power in the form of NADH or NADPH. The normal response to oxidant toxins is via the hexose phosphate shunt, which has reducing mechanisms to maintain glutathione in the reduced state.

Some oxidizing agents denature hemoglobin directly, resulting in precipitates known as *Heinz bodies*. Heinz bodies appear within 24 hours of exposure to the offending agent and may occur with or without methemoglobinemia. In addition, oxidative injury to the cell membrane may occur. Both Heinz body formation and membrane damage are irreversible and alter the deformability of the red cell. The Heinz bodies are seen with Wright-Giemsa stain as a single round colorless inclusion sometimes bulging from the red cell membrane and encompassing about one-fifth of the red cell diameter. New methylene blue stains Heinz bodies blue. The spleen functions to remove inclusions such as these from red cells, so if the spleen is absent, these remain longer. The spleen of the cat is less able to remove inclusions from red cells, so a few Heinz bodies are often present in the blood of normal cats. The cat also is particularly prone to hemolysis after exposure to oxidants because cats have more sulfhydryl groups on their hemoglobin molecule susceptible to oxidation. The cat also lacks the enzyme glucuronyl transferase, which is needed to conjugate certain potentially toxic drugs for excretion.

Clinical Signs

Signs of acute hypoxia occur when >40% of the hemoglobin is converted to methemoglobin. Methemoglobinemia imparts a chocolate brown color to the blood. In some cases, this can be dramatic and obvious as the blood is drawn. Mucous membranes have a cyanotic or blue-brown color and the patient is dyspneic despite the lack of clinical or radiographic evidence of heart or lung dysfunction.

Heinz body anemia may result from a combination of extravascular and intravascular hemolysis. In severe toxicity, edema of the face may occur. The exact cause of the edema is not clear, but might reflect acute cardiac decompensation because of hypoxia.

Causes of Oxidative Toxicity

In humans, an inherited deficiency of methemoglobin reductase or G6PD results in increased susceptibility to methemoglobinemia or Heinz body anemia. Although methemoglobin reductase deficiency has been found in dogs, most cases in animals are caused by an ingestion of toxins. One of the first descriptions of Heinz body ane-

mia in cats was associated with the use of methylene blue as a urinary antiseptic. Affected cats developed severe hemolysis that resolved when the drug was stopped. Acetaminophen causes Heinz body anemia with methemoglobinemia in cats. This toxicity is common as well-meaning owners give the drug to their cats, and as little as one-half tablet (163 mg) may result in signs of toxicity. Because cats are unable to metabolize and excrete the drug like other species, the half-life of the drug is prolonged, making it even more toxic. Methemoglobinemia and severe intravascular and extravascular hemolysis, often with facial edema, occur. In addition, acetaminophen causes necrosis of the liver in cats, further increasing morbidity and mortality. Other toxins reported to cause oxidative toxicity in cats include benzocaine used as a local anesthetic on the skin or sprayed into the pharynx of an anesthetized cat to facilitate tracheal intubation. DL-Methionine, a urinary acidifier, and propofol, an anesthetic, also cause oxidant damage to feline red cells.

Ingestion of onions causes Heinz body anemia in cattle, horses, dogs, and cats. Onions contain *n*-propyl disulfide, which decreases G6PD activity in red cells and inhibits the production of reduced glutathione. In addition, acetaminophen (in higher doses than used for cats), naphthalene (mothballs), and benzocaine have been associated with hemolysis in dogs.

Nitrate poisoning can be a serious problem in cattle. Sources include contaminated water or feeds such as Sudan grass. The nitrate is converted to nitrite by rumen flora. The absorbed nitrite is an active oxidant and causes methemoglobinemia. Toxicity from ingesting red maple leaves or treatment with phenothiazine causes oxidant hemolysis in horses.

Copper or Zinc Toxicity

The mechanism of copper and zinc toxicity is not well understood but appears to be primarily oxidant damage, along with some inhibition of glycolytic enzymes. Methemoglobinemia is sometimes present in poisoned animals. Sheep seem to be especially sensitive to hemolysis caused by copper accumulating in the liver from contamination of forage. Copper is toxic to the liver and in times of stress, release of copper into the blood may cause severe intravascular hemolysis. Although the copper accumulation is gradual, the hemolytic crisis is acute and may occur when the pastures become dry in the fall. Copper sulfate placed in ponds to kill algae may poison livestock.

An inherited disease similar to human Wilson's disease is prevalent in Bedlington terriers. Copper is stored in the liver even when intake in the diet is not excessive. This results in progressive liver failure leading to cirrhosis. Hemolysis is uncommon.

Zinc toxicity is most commonly seen in young dogs ingesting zinc-containing foreign bodies such as pennies. Prior to 1982, pennies were composed of copper; after that zinc was used. The result is acute intravascular hemolysis that subsides if the foreign bodies are removed.

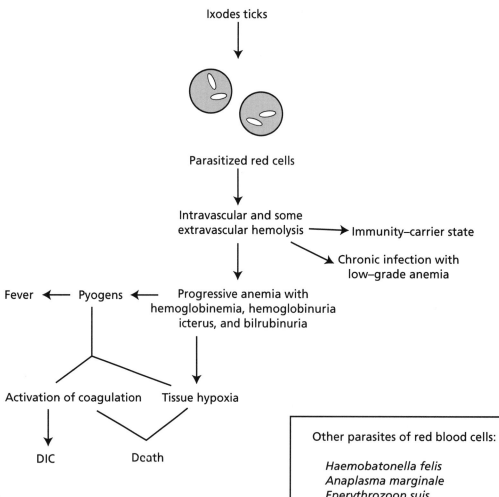

Pathogenesis of Babesiosis

Ixodes ticks

Parasitized red cells

Intravascular and some extravascular hemolysis → Immunity–carrier state

→ Chronic infection with low–grade anemia

Fever ← Pyogens ← Progressive anemia with hemoglobinemia, hemoglobinuria icterus, and bilrubinuria

Activation of coagulation   Tissue hypoxia

DIC   Death

Other parasites of red blood cells:

Haemobatonella felis
Anaplasma marginale
Eperythrozoon suis

Bacterial Infections

Leptospirosis is a contagious disease of animals and humans caused by spirochetes of several serovars, most of which are subgroups of *Leptospira interrogans*. Organisms are shed in the urine of infected patients and may survive in water for long periods of time. In calves and occasionally in lambs, the *pomona* serovar causes icterus and intravascular hemolysis. Hemolysis occurs much less often in adult cattle, dogs or horses.

Bacillary hemoglobinuria (Red Water Disease) is an acute disease of cattle caused by *Clostridium hemolyticum*. The disease occurs in the western United States and is characterized by fever, intravascular hemolysis with hemoglobinuria, and sometimes icterus. The organism produces a toxin that causes hemolysis and hepatic necrosis and DIC. The most typical lesions at necropsy are pale hemorrhagic infarcts of the liver, caused by thrombosis of the portal vein. Other hemolytic disorders of cattle are anaplasmosis, babesiosis, postparturient hemoglobinuria, leptospirosis, and toxicity from water, kale, copper, and onions.

Equine Infectious Anemia (EIA)

The cause of EIA, sometimes called *swamp fever,* is a lentivirus that is a subgroup of retroviruses. The virus is transmitted primarily by biting flies that can harbor live virus for up to one hour. If another horse is bitten during that time, it can become infected. The virus also is readily transmitted by blood-contaminated needles, by transfusion, and transplacentally. Less than 1 mL of blood is required for transfer of infection from one horse to another.

The clinical disease is variable. The acute form is characterized by fever, sometimes with edema, whereas subacute or chronic forms are characterized by weight loss, splenomegaly, fever, edema, and anemia, in recurring cycles. The anemia is difficult to classify and probably includes hemolysis and decreased production of red cells by the marrow. The immune response to the virus causes immune complexes and vasculitis. Infection persists in the white blood cells for the life of the horse, but clinical signs are intermittent. Diagnosis is made by detection of antibody with an agar gel immunodiffusion test sometimes called a Coggins test.

Parasites of Red Blood Cells

Any disease caused by a red cell parasite is more likely to occur in splenectomized animals since the spleen is the major defense against these organisms. As a general rule, large red cell parasites like *Babesia* and *Plasmodium* are likely to cause intravascular hemolysis, whereas small parasites like *Haemorbartonella, Eperythrozoon* and *Anaplasma* attach to the outside of the red cell membrane. They may dislodge in stored blood, so blood should be examined immediately.

Babesiosis spread by ticks, affects humans, cattle, sheep and goats, pigs, horses, and dogs in various parts of the world (**Figure**). Infections generally do not spread between species. Babesiosis of cattle caused by *Babesia bigemina* was the cause of Texas fever, the first disease of humans or animals in which an arthropod was proved to be a vector. The disease was controlled by eliminating the tick vector, leading the way for control of human diseases such as malaria and yellow fever. Babesiosis is serious in situations where cattle are moved from a nonendemic to an endemic area because these animals have not acquired resistance by constant exposure. Clinical signs include hemoglobinemia and hemoglobinuria with fever and regenerative anemia. Infections vary from fulminating and rapidly fatal to chronic or inapparent. Organisms may be seen in the red cells, and serological tests are available. Most U.S. cases in dogs have occurred in the southern states, with young dogs being most susceptible. A high prevalence of infection has been recognized in racing greyhounds, some of which have traveled extensively. *Babesia* parasites are spread by the same tick that causes ehrlichiosis, so coinfections commonly occur in dogs.

Malaria caused by *Plasmodium* species is one of the most important diseases worldwide in humans and is also seen in birds and nonhuman primates. The disease sometimes is called *blackwater fever* because of hemoglobinuria. Malaria has been eliminated in many parts of the world through mosquito control, but where it is still endemic, organisms have developed resistance to some antimalarial drugs.

Hemobartonellosis, also called *feline infectious anemia*, occurs primarily as an opportunistic infection in cats immunosuppressed from some other primary illness. In blood smears stained with Wright-Giemsa stain, the organisms may resemble rods, cocci, or rings. They may be single or in groups on the surface of red cells. On new methylene blue stain organisms cannot be distinguished from punctate reticulocytes. Attachment of organisms to the red cell membrane causes erosions that predispose to hemolysis, either by direct fragility or by immune-mediated mechanisms.

The natural mode of transmission has not been established, but fleas or ticks are suspected to be the vectors. Cats appear to become chronic carriers after primary infection, although organisms are not always present in the blood. Hemolysis is not necessarily part of the carrier state.

Transient fever is the first sign and is followed by hemolytic anemia usually with organisms visible on red cells. Icterus may be seen with increased bilirubin and urobilinogen concentrations in the urine. Splenomegaly is common.

Eperythrozoonosis causes hemolytic anemia with fever in young swine, mainly in midwestern and southern states. These parasites resemble *Haemobartonella* and the mechanism of hemolysis and findings on the hemogram are the same.

Anaplasmosis is a common debilitating disease of cattle causing fever, anemia, icterus, and emaciation. Ticks are biological vectors, but mechanical transmission occurs as well by biting flies or injections with contaminated needles. Young animals are rarely severely affected, but severe signs occur when exposure occurs after >3 years of age and mortality may be >50% in this group.

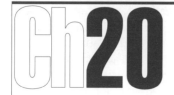

Other Causes of Hemolysis

Red Cells Damaged by Passage Through Fibrin,
as seen in Microangiopathic Hemolysis

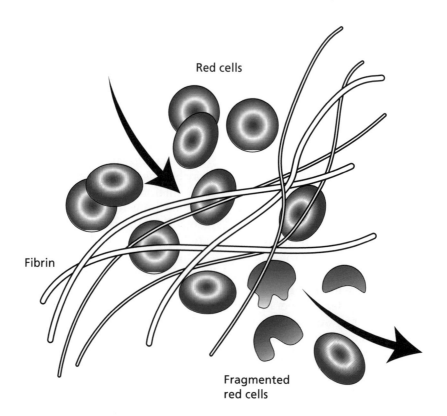

Red cells

Fibrin

Fragmented
red cells

Toxins

Certain drugs and toxins cause hemolysis by immune-mediated mechanisms. Vaccination, especially with modified live-virus vaccines, has been implicated as a cause of IMHA in dogs. Other drugs linked to IMHA in dogs are levamisole and some antibiotics, especially cephalosporins and sulfonamides. Cats rarely develop primary IMHA but have developed Coombs positive hemolytic anemia when treated for hyperthyroidism with propylthiouracil, or less commonly with methimazole.

Many toxins including acetaminophen, onions, and red maple leaves, cause hemolysis by an oxidative mechanism (*see* Chapter 17). Water toxicity has been reported in calves that overdrink when provided with unlimited water. Freshwater drowning in any species causes rapid intravascular hemolysis. The cause in both of these situations is an osmotic imbalance caused by rapid absorption of water from the intestines or lungs. Certain snake and spider venoms may cause hemolytic anemia with local pain, swelling or necrosis, and thrombosis and circulatory collapse.

Metabolic Causes

Postparturient hemoglobinuria from hemolysis occurs in high-producing dairy cattle during the first few weeks after parturition. The cause appears to be hypophosphatemia, which occurs when losses in the milk exceed intake. In severe hypophosphatemia, red cell glycolysis is impeded causing decreased 2,3-DPG and ATP production and shortened red cell life span. A similar mechanism of hemolysis has occurred in dogs or cats within 12–24 hours after initiation of insulin treatment for severe diabetes mellitus. Insulin promotes a shift of phosphorus from the extracellular to the intracellular space, resulting in a drop in the circulating concentration of phosphorus. Signs of hemolysis occur only after severe drops in phosphorus, usually <1 mg/dL.

Splenomegaly can occur for many reasons, but whenever the spleen is very large, it can remove blood cells at an excessive rate. This condition, called *hypersplenism*, can cause premature removal of not only red cells, but also platelets and white cells.

Microangiopathic (Traumatic) Hemolysis

Microangiopathic hemolysis is a form of intravascular hemolysis associated with physical trauma to red cells as they pass through areas of turbulent blood flow. The cells break by smashing into rigid obstructions in their path. Microangiopathic hemolysis may be seen in dogs with severe heartworm disease, especially when large masses of worms obstruct the vena cava. Tumors with abnormal and torturous blood vessels, usually hemangiosarcomas but occasionally large hemangiomas, cause hemolysis in dogs and occasionally in cats.

Splenic torsion occurs in some deep-chested breeds of dogs. When the spleen twists, thin-walled veins become obstructed before the arteries and red cells are damaged as they are pushed through the partially obstructed veins.

Traumatic rupture of red cells occurs when red cells pass through regions of intravascular coagulation. Although blood does not normally clot in the vascular tree, conditions such as DIC or thrombosis or embolism cause red cells to become damaged as they pass through a mesh of fibrin strands (*see* Chapter 49).

Rarely traumatic hemolysis has been seen in human (and potentially animal) athletes after prolonged running or walking. In this situation, red cells are damaged as they pass through the capillaries of the feet.

The characteristic finding on a blood smear in a patient with microangiopathic hemolysis is fragmentation of red cells, referred to as *schistocytes* (**Figure**). They may take the form of helmets, triangles, or small spherocytes. Since the hemolysis is intravascular, hemoglobinemia and hemoglobinuria would be expected findings as well. However, if the degree of hemolysis is small, as is usually the case, the free hemoglobin may be bound to haptoglobin and removed to extravascular sites for metabolism, and the only findings might be a mild regenerative anemia.

Inherited Red Cell Defects

Most known inherited red cell disorders of animals involve defects in the Embden-Meyerhof pathway (*see* Chapter 5, Part B). Since the mature red cell has no nucleus, it relies on anaerobic metabolism for the production of ATP for energy needed for survival. The severity of the anemia depends on the site of the pathway disrupted and the degree of the disruption. Causes of inherited hemolytic anemia include red cell enzyme deficiencies, membrane abnormalities, or abnormal hemoglobin.

Pyruvate kinase (PK) deficiency has been reported in Basenjis, beagles, and several other breeds of dogs, and Abyssinian cats. Red cells have a short life span because they are unable to generate enough ATP. Affected puppies have reduced exercise tolerance but grow normally. Reticulocytosis and splenomegaly from extramedullary hematopoiesis are present. This disease tends to be progressive, and finally myelofibrosis develops.

Phosphofructokinase deficiency has been found primarily in English springer spaniels. Acute hemolytic episodes occur after excitement or exercise. Hyperventilation and respiratory alkalosis predispose the sensitive red cells to hemolysis. Because of a similar defect in skeletal muscle, weakness and collapse may occur. Episodes are periodic with spontaneous recovery.

Porphyria is the only hemoglobinopathy known to occur in animals (*see* Chapter 6). Because of a failure to produce adequate amounts of porphyrinogens for hemoglobin synthesis, affected individuals accumulate useless porphyrins. The teeth and urine fluoresce under ultraviolet light, but measurement of increased levels of urinary uroporphyrins confirms the diagnosis.

Nonregenerative Anemia

Causes of Nonregenerative Anemia

Acute blood loss or hemolysis (first 3-4 days)

Anemia of chronic disease or in inflammation

Chronic renal failure

Deficiencies (rare)
    Folate, cobalamin, iron (usually regenerative)
    Malnutrition

Metabolic diseases
    Hypothyroidism, other endocrine deficiencies
    Hyperestrogenism (Iatrogenic or neoplasia)
    Liver disease

Infections
    Retrovirus infection
    Ehrlichiosis
    Parvovirus infection

Drugs / toxins

Radiation

Pure red cell aplasia
    Most immune mediated
    Idiopathic

Aplastic anemia
    Infections, drugs, toxins
    Immune mediated
    Idiopathic

Necrosis or sclerosis of the marrow

Myelofibrosis

Myelodysplasia

Acute lymphoblastic or acute myelogenous leukemia

Myeloma

Malignant histiocytosis

Other malignancy

Nonregenerative anemia usually has a gradual onset, and is often severe by the time the patient first becomes symptomatic. Compensatory mechanisms to improve oxygenation of tissues such as increased heart and respiratory rates are in place. Most species will also have an increased concentration of red cell 2,3-DPG, which aids in the delivery of oxygen to the tissues. Species such as cats and cattle lack this enzyme, but the same effect of unloading oxygen is chloride dependent. If an animal loses >50% of its red cell volume acutely, one would expect obvious clinical signs related to hemorrhage or hemolysis, whereas if this same loss occurred from a decreased production of red cells, clinical signs would be minimal or absent. Another clue that an anemia might be nonregenerative is concurrent leukopenia or thrombocytopenia, or both (pancytopenia), indicative of damage to the marrow.

The anemia is usually normocytic and normochromic, with an absolute reticulocyte count of <60,000/μL or a corrected reticulocyte percentage of <1%. Nonregenerative anemia may be macrocytic in some cats with anemia secondary to feline leukemia virus (FeLV) or myelodysplasia (see Chapters 24 and 26), and rarely in dogs with exposure to certain toxins or with deficiencies.

Nucleated red cells may be present in the blood of anemic patients regardless of whether or not an anemia is regenerative. One must avoid the temptation to consider circulating nucleated red cells as "immature" cells indicative of an active marrow response. In the presence of nonregenerative anemia, circulating nucleated red cells are indicative of marrow damage, dysfunction, or malignancy.

Nonregenerative anemia can be caused by exogenous factors affecting the marrow or by primary marrow failure (Figure). If stem cells, hematopoietic growth factors, or other nutritional components are inadequate, or if suppressive or toxic factors such as drugs, autoantibodies affecting progenitors, or substances secreted by leukemic cells are present, adequate numbers of normally functioning red cells cannot be produced.

Animals with any debilitating or chronic illness commonly have a mild anemia, known as anemia of chronic disease or inflammation. In cats, nonregenerative anemia also occurs secondary to infection with retroviruses.

Pure Red Cell Aplasia

Pure red cell aplasia is defined as a nonregenerative, normocytic normochromic anemia with a selective reduction of erythroid precursors in the marrow. The most common cause in dogs is probably immune mediated, whereas in cats, it is probably FeLV infection.

Most immune-mediated destruction of red cells occurs within the peripheral circulation. Some cases are so acute that sufficient time (3–4 days) has not elapsed to allow for reticulocytosis. In other cases, reticulocytes and even earlier red cell precursors are destroyed in the marrow. These patients may have a gradual onset of nor-

mocytic normochromic nonregenerative anemia. The bone marrow may show erythroid hypoplasia or evidence of intramedullary destruction of cells (erythrophagocytosis). Increased numbers of lymphocytes and plasma cells may be present, implying an immune response.

Diagnosis of the nonregenerative form of IMHA may be relatively easy if the Coombs' test result is positive or if spherocytosis is present, but in other cases the diagnosis is made only by excluding other causes of nonregenerative anemia.

Pancytopenia

Pancytopenia is defined as a decrease in red cells, granulocytes, and platelets in the blood. It is a descriptive term only and not a diagnosis; however, whenever all 3 cell lines are suppressed, the source of the abnormality is in the bone marrow. The marrow may have a primary intrinsic abnormality or may be damaged by an extrinsic problem. These causes are discussed in Chapter 26. *Aplastic anemia* is defined as pancytopenia with decreased production of all 3 cell lines in the marrow and replacement with fat. With aplastic anemia, typically <25% of the marrow is composed of hematopoietic cells.

Many disease processes can interfere temporarily or permanently with the viability of the pluripotent stem cell, resulting in aplastic anemia. Affected animals are at risk for bacterial sepsis from granulocytopenia or bleeding from thrombocytopenia. In most cases, neutropenia occurs first, then thrombocytopenia, and finally anemia. The Hct may fall more quickly if significant bleeding occurs. Some lymphocytes may persist in the blood and marrow, but often lymphopenia is present as well, with only long-lived memory cells surviving.

When faced with a patient with nonregenerative anemia, one would first search for causes extrinsic to the marrow, such as exposure to drugs or toxins; renal disease; other chronic illnesses; endocrine, nutritional, or immune-mediated factors. If none is found, then the marrow is examined. If pancytopenia is present, both aspiration to obtain specimens for detailed cytological examination and a core biopsy to determine cellularity and look for fibrosis must be done.

Prognosis

Nonregenerative anemias often have a worse prognosis than do regenerative anemias. However, nonregenerative anemia secondary to renal failure, immune-mediated causes, metabolic or deficiency diseases, or a treatable chronic illness may be fully reversible since the marrow in each is normal. When the marrow has been damaged by drugs, toxins, infectious agents, or radiation, the anemia may be irreversible. Just as the onset of the nonregenerative form of IMHA can have a slow, insidious onset, the response to treatment also can be slow. Red cell precursors must be restored before the Hct can rise, and this may take 1–2 weeks or longer if antibody persists.

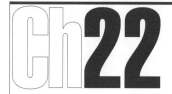

Anemia of Chronic Disease/ Anemia of Inflammatory Disease

Sequestration of Iron in Macrophages in Anemia of Chronic Disease

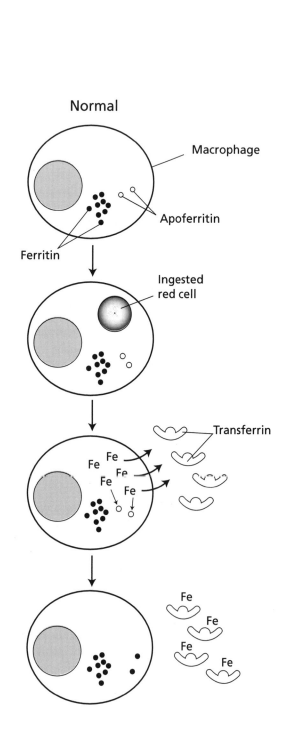

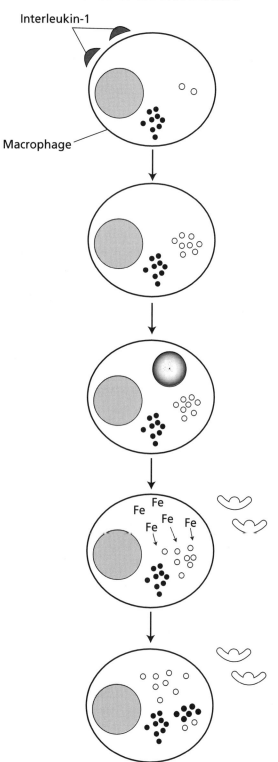

A common cause of anemia in dogs and cats is anemia of chronic disease that accompanies infection, neoplasia, and other debilitating diseases. Despite the fact that it occurs so commonly, it is of relatively little clinical significance because it is rarely severe enough to cause clinical signs. However, it probably has been treated by more unneeded and ineffective hematinics and vitamins than any other anemia. It is important to recognize the occurrence of this condition, put it into perspective, and move on to the more important task of diagnosis and treatment of the underlying disease. The anemia develops slowly over 2–3 weeks but remains mild, with the Hct seldom dropping to <25% in dogs. Because feline red cells have a shorter life span than those of dogs, the Hct may drop more quickly and to a greater degree in cats, but usually remains >20%. More severe anemia means another cause must be sought. Anemia of chronic disease may be superimposed on another cause of anemia. The anemia is usually normocytic normochromic, but in rare cases may be microcytic and hypochromic, leading to confusion with iron deficiency. Generally, the abnormalities associated with the underlying disease overshadow the anemia, which is often asymptomatic.

In Chronic Disease

Several factors are involved in the pathogenesis of anemia of chronic disease. Cytokines are a family of peptides that include interleukins, interferons, tumor necrosis factor, and certain hematopoietic growth factors. They are secreted by fibroblasts, endothelial cells, lymphocytes, macrophages, and some hematopoietic cells in response to infections and other tissue injury. Some cytokines as well as bacterial by-products such as endotoxin can inhibit erythropoiesis.

Chronic diseases are associated with impairment of the transfer of storage iron from macrophages back to hematopoietic tissue. Normally iron is released into the plasma, bound to transferrin, and transported back to the marrow to be incorporated into newly developing red cell precursors. Since 95% of the iron used for red cell production comes from reutilization of senescent red cell iron, a delay in the release of iron from macrophages limits the availability of iron. The sequestered iron is taken up by apoferritin, which is synthesized by macrophages to form ferritin, the storage form of iron (**Figure**). Ferritin consists of a core of ferric hydroxide encased in apoferritin, a protein shell. Excessive iron remains in the marrow, and the serum ferritin level is normal to high, especially in dogs. Serum ferritin concentrations correlate reasonably well with total body stores of iron, and species-specific assays have been validated for use in dogs but are not readily available for clinical practice. Serum iron is decreased in anemia of chronic disease, and the iron saturation of transferrin is low to normal. The iron-binding capacity (transferrin) does not increase. This is helpful in differentiating anemia of chronic disease from iron deficiency anemia. Secretion of erythropoietin is decreased as well as the response to erythropoietin of committed red cell progenitors, BFU-Es and CFU-Es. Red cells that are produced have a shortened survival time, possibly because of increased uptake of red cells by activated macrophages in the spleen. An immune mechanism also may be involved in decreased red cell survival, as the presence of IgG has been noted on red cells, leading to increased phagocytosis by macrophages.

Whether this decrease in serum iron is beneficial to the patient is not clear. It has been suggested that part of the pathogenicity of bacteria is to compete with the host for iron, and by making iron unavailable to the bacteria, the host can overcome the infection. If this decrease in iron does play a role in the elimination of pathogenic bacteria, it is probably a minor one.

In Inflammation

In the presence of inflammation, dogs can develop anemia after 2–3 weeks, whereas in cats, the Hct decreases significantly over 7–10 days. In cats, serum iron concentrations decrease over the same time period and erythropoietin concentrations do not increase. Although a shortened red cell life span is thought to be the major cause of the initial drop in Hct, it obviously is not the only cause because an appropriate erythropoietin and reticulocyte response fails to develop, thus inhibiting an expected marrow response to the red cell destruction.

The cause of anemia of chronic disease may be multifactorial, depending on both the underlying disease and other superimposed factors such as malnutrition, chronic blood loss through repeated blood sampling or gastrointestinal losses, renal failure, consumption coagulopathy, drugs used in treatment, or even marrow infiltration with malignant cells.

If the anemia is severe, an additional cause is likely to be present, as typically the Hct in anemia of chronic disease ranges from the low end of the reference range to 10%–15% below it, and is rarely severe enough to cause clinical signs. Specific treatment of anemia of chronic disease is neither necessary nor beneficial. Iron supplementation should not be used. If the underlying disease is reversible, the Hct will return to normal.

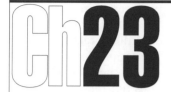

Ch23 Anemia Secondary to Renal or Endocrine Disease

Reasons for Anemia of Renal Failure

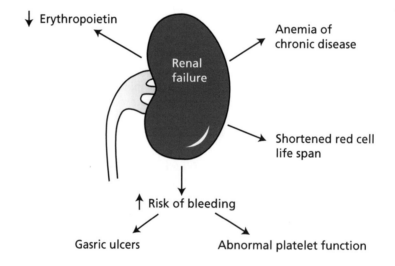

↓ Erythropoietin

Anemia of chronic disease

Renal failure

Shortened red cell life span

↑ Risk of bleeding

Gasric ulcers

Abnormal platelet function

Anemia Secondary to Renal Disease

Erythropoietin is produced normally by peritubular endothelial cells in the renal cortex at a rate inversely proportional to the oxygen content of the blood. It most effectively stimulates the later committed erythroid progenitors, CFU-Es, and at higher concentrations also stimulates the earlier BFU-Es. When renal failure becomes chronic, production of erythropoietin decreases and anemia ensues. The anemia is normocytic, normochromic, and nonregenerative. Erythropoietin concentration may be low or normal in an anemic animal when one would expect the appropriate response to be an increased concentration. The presence or absence of anemia can be a clue in determining whether renal failure is acute or chronic. In some animals, especially in cats, the clinical signs of anemia rather than those of renal failure may be the reason why the patient is presented to the veterinarian. In a survey of feline red cell transfusions given at Tufts University, renal failure was one of the most common reasons for transfusion.

Chronically azotemic patients may become anemic for additional reasons (**Figure**). Although decreased erythropoietin is most significant, coexisting problems are decreased life span of red cells, anemia of chronic disease, a poorly defined defect in platelet function, and blood loss from gastric ulcers, which commonly occur secondary to renal failure. Blood urea nitrogen (BUN) elevated disproportionately to creatinine could be an indication of gastrointestinal blood loss, as digested red cells are absorbed and metabolized with urea as a by-product. Proposed causes of decreased red cell survival include decreased utilization of the hexose monophosphate shunt resulting in oxidative damage to red cells, and toxic effects of urea, phenols, and other retained substances. The oxidative damage to feline red cells may be evident by the presence of Heinz bodies. A protective effect of the retention of phosphorus in renal failure is the increase in 2,3-DPG in dogs, which improves oxygen delivery to tissues despite a reduced red cell mass.

Treatment with recombinant erythropoietin has been of significant benefit to human patients with chronic renal failure. Although progression of renal failure continues, the quality of life improves as the need for red cell transfusions is removed. Recombinant human erythropoietin (r-HuEPO, Epogen-Amgen, Thousand Oaks, CA) also has been used with some success in comparable canine and feline patients. The structures of erythropoietins in these species are similar but not identical to that in humans. When dogs and cats are treated with r-HuEPO, reticulocytosis is usually evident by the end of the first week, and the Hct rises within 3–4 weeks. Because of increased demands on the marrow for erythropoiesis, iron supplementation is indicated at least until the Hct is stabilized. Decreased concentrations of serum iron have been documented in approximately 30% of patients receiving erythropoietin. Iron supplementation usually is given in the form of oral ferrous sulfate. Since iron can irritate the stomach, patients must be monitored carefully. Because of species differences in erythropoietin and because r-HuEPO is suspended in human albumin, allergic reactions or antierythropoietin antibodies may develop in up to 50% of dogs and cats any time from 4 weeks to several months into treatment, and require the treatment to be stopped. Because antibodies also react against endogenous erythropoietin, the anemia can become more severe than it was prior to treatment. Long-term transfusion therapy may be required in these patients. Sometimes the antibodies decline over time, but repeated therapy is less likely to be successful.

Administration of H_2 blockers such as cimetidine and ranitidine helps to minimize the risk of additional blood loss through ulceration of the gastrointestinal tract.

Anemia Secondary to Endocrine Disorders

Nonregenerative anemia also can occur with endogenous or exogenous hyperestrogenism, but is associated with marrow stem cell damage and is discussed in Chapter 25.

Hypothyroidism causes a mild anemia in humans and dogs, probably because of a physiological adaptation to decreased oxygen consumption and decreased metabolic rate. It has been estimated that 30%–50% of hypothyroid dogs have Hct values below the reference range. Circulating target cells may be present. These cells have excessive membrane, probably because of increased cholesterol deposition. Target cells have a red membrane and a colorless halo around a red center and are also seen in animals with abnormal cholesterol because of liver disease, or after splenectomy. Normally the spleen functions to remove excessive membrane. The anemia of hypothyroidism is mild and asymptomatic and resolves with thyroid supplementation.

Other endocrine disorders that might be associated with mild anemia are hypopituitarism, hypoadrenocorticism, and decreased growth hormone. Pregnancy commonly has been associated with a decrease in Hct. This decrease is caused by an increase in plasma volume, however, and the red cell mass remains normal.

Folate Absorption and Metabolism

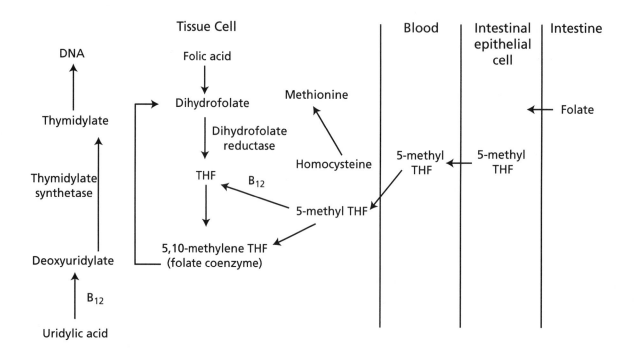

Folate is required for the synthesis of 3 of the 4 base pairs in DNA. The vitamin is initially inert and is activated via dehydrofolate (DHF) reductase to tetrahydrofolate (THF) and is then incorporated into nucleic acid (see **Figure**). Folate absorbed by the intestine is converted to 5-methyl THF in the intestinal epithelial cells and secreted into the plasma in that form. When it is taken up by tissue cells, including erythroid precursors, THF serves as a source of 5,10-methylene THF, which is the coenzyme needed to produce thymidylate used in DNA synthesis.

Within the cells, the folate cycle also involves conversion of DHF to THF by DHF reductase. Cobalamin functions in folate metabolism in the production of folate coenzyme. A deficiency of cobalamin leads to impaired conversion of homocysteine to methionine, the trapping of folate as 5-methyl THF, and ultimately impaired synthesis of DNA. The marrow is significantly affected by inhibition of DNA synthesis. In most tissues, cell division occurs only as needed for repair, whereas hematopoietic cells are dividing constantly. All cell lines of the marrow are affected, but morphological changes are most evident in erythroid precursors. The granulocytic precursors also are affected, resulting in giant band neutrophils or hypersegmented neutrophils. Despite the decrease in DNA synthesis, the synthesis of RNA and proteins remains normal. Asynchrony of maturation (megaloblastosis) occurs in that the nucleus of erythroid precursors matures more slowly than does the cytoplasm. Skipped mitoses result in enlarged mature red cells and an increased MCV.

Because of the abnormality in production, some precursors do not survive the development process and die while still in the marrow. The end result is ineffective hematopoiesis, seen in the blood as variable combinations of anemia, neutropenia, and thrombocytopenia.

In humans a deficiency of cobalamin usually is caused by a lack of gastric production of intrinsic factor and is called *pernicious anemia*. Intrinsic factor, in the presence of an increased pH in the duodenum, attaches to cobalamin and subsequently to specific receptors on mucosal cells in the ileum, allowing for absorption. In dogs, cats, and perhaps other animals, intrinsic factor is produced in the pancreas rather than the stomach. True pernicious anemia due to a lack of gastric intrinsic factor has not been found in animals. In ruminants, the rumen flora produce all the needed cobalamin. The same is true of flora in the cecum of horses.

Folate is present in most foods and synthesized by intestinal bacteria so nutritional deficiency is rare. Cobalamin is also present in the normal dog or cat diet. Folate and cobalamin deficiencies have been produced by feeding artificial diets to dogs and cats. Anemia from folate deficiency can occur after 2–4 months in dogs, but a much longer period is required for clinical signs of cobalamin deficiency to appear because of prolonged hepatic storage. The anemia in both deficiencies is not overtly macrocytic in dogs as described in humans. Instead it is normocytic normochromic, with some macrocytes seen on blood smears and megaloblastosis in the marrow.

Abnormalities in folate or cobalamin concentrations have been documented in certain maldigestion, malabsorption, or bacterial overgrowth syndromes in dogs and cats. Only severe chronic cases of malabsorption or exocrine pancreatic insufficiency (EP) result in folate or cobalamin deficiency. The lack of intrinsic factor in EPI may contribute to the finding of low cobalamin concentrations, since concentrations remain low even after enzyme replacement therapy. Folate may be increased in EPI because of enhanced absorption secondary to decreased intestinal pH. In dogs with intestinal bacterial overgrowth, cobalamin may be decreased because of bacterial utilization, and folate increased because of production by bacteria. Anemia is not present in these situations unless the condition is severe and prolonged. Diagnosis is by finding decreased serum folate or cobalamin concentrations. Successful treatment of the underlying disease would allow folate or cobalamin concentrations to normalize; however, supplementation can be used for severe deficiencies.

An autosomal recessive inherited malabsorption of cobalamin has been described in giant Schnauzers and border collies. This rare defect is caused by an absence of the receptor for the intrinsic factor–cobalamin complex in the ileal brush border. A chronic nonregenerative anemia and neutropenia are present. Treatment is parenteral cobalamin given intermittently for life.

Certain chemotherapeutic drugs inhibit folate. The anticancer drug methotrexate inhibits DHF reductase and at high doses can cause megaloblastic anemia (**Figure**). Hydroxyurea, which inhibits DNA synthesis, causes a mild to moderate macrocytic anemia in dogs and humans. This anemia, which is evident by megaloblastic changes in the marrow, resembles the anemia of folate or cobalamin deficiency but is not associated with a decrease in either.

Megaloblastic anemia occasionally has been seen in dogs treated with trimethoprim-sulfa combinations, fenbendazole, quinidine, or the anticonvulsive agents primidone, diphenylhydantoin, or phenobarbital.

Macrocytic nonregenerative anemia occurs in cats with FeLV infection and in dogs or cats with myelodysplasia (*see* Chapters 24 and 54). Here skipped mitoses and ineffective hematopoiesis are the probable mechanisms. Treatment of these patients with folate or cobalamin is of no benefit since serum concentrations are normal. Macrocytosis is seen as an inherited condition in some families of poodles. These dogs have MCVs ranging from 85 to 95 fL (normal, 60–77 fL) but are not anemic and have no clinical signs of illness even though some megaloblastosis is present in the marrow. No treatment is indicated.

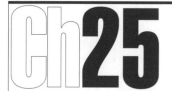

Infectious Causes
of Nonregenerative Anemia

Mechanisms of Anemia Caused by Feline Leukemia Virus

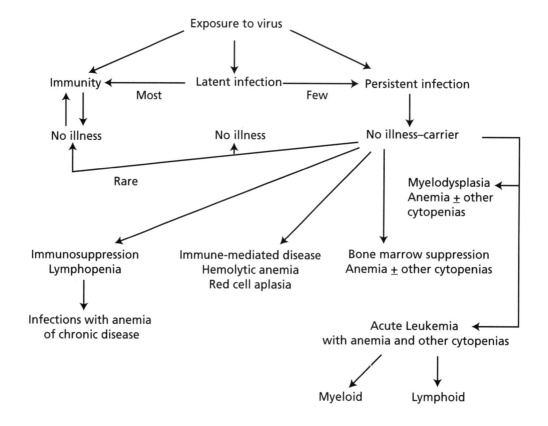

Feline Leukemia Virus

FeLV, in the oncornavirus subgroup of retroviruses, commonly causes a severe, usually nonregenerative anemia that may be macrocytic or normocytic and normochromic. Whenever macrocytic anemia occurs without reticulocytosis in a cat, FeLV infection should be suspected. Macrocytosis often is associated with abnormalities in the marrow (myelodysplasia). Severe nonregenerative anemia occurs to a lesser extent with feline immunodeficiency virus (FIV) infection. Also a retrovirus, FIV is classified in the lentivirus subgroup, as is the human immunodeficiency virus (HIV). If anemia does occur with FIV, it is more likely to be mild and may be secondary to something else (anemia of chronic disease). FIV is more likely to suppress granulocytic than erythroid progenitors.

Retroviruses cause anemia by several mechanisms (**Figure**). The virus can directly suppress the marrow. Anemia can also be secondary to coexisting marrow abnormalities such as fibrosis, dysplasia, or leukemia, or even complicated by anemia of chronic disease. Essentially FeLV can affect any or all hematopoietic cell lines and cause suppression (cytopenias), abnormal maturation, or malignant transformation of myeloid erythroid, and lymphoid cell lines (see Chapter 52). In past years, approximately 70% of anemic cats (Hct <20%) were FeLV antigen positive. This was equivalent to the frequency of cats diagnosed with lymphoma and leukemia testing positive for FeLV. That percentage has declined along with the overall prevalence of FeLV in North America. The overall incidence of anemia probably has decreased as well, although current epidemiological studies have not been done.

The pathogenesis of FeLV-associated anemia is complex. The 3 subgroups (A, B, and C) have different effects in experimentally infected kittens. Subgroup A causes a transient macrocytic anemia with a regenerative marrow response; subgroup B does not cause any disease. Subgroup C, which like B arises from A by recombination with endogenous feline gene sequences, induces fatal red cell aplasia or aplastic anemia. Subgroup C also has been associated with naturally occurring nonregenerative anemia in cats. The mechanism of impairment of hematopoiesis may be direct inhibition of erythroid progenitors by viral gene products, or interaction with lymphoreticular cells, especially T cells, that normally produce the necessary hematopoietic growth factors. Since FeLV infects erythroid progenitors, it is also possible that a host immunopathological response against infected cells causes their destruction, but evidence for this is lacking.

When presented with an FeLV-positive cat with nonregenerative anemia, one must first search for other coexisting systemic problems such as infections secondary to immunosuppression, or primary marrow problems such as myelodysplasia or leukemic infiltration. Successful treatment of coexisting problems may result in spontaneous improvement in the anemia. Many FeLV-positive anemic cats have circulating nucleated red cells, even though the minority show evidence of reticulocytosis.

Many FeLV-positive anemic cats die or are euthanized because of refractory anemia, a few develop leukemia or myelodysplasia, and a few will recover. Reasons for euthanasia include concerns about prognosis, cost of treatment, or danger to other household cats. Some cats appear to respond to corticosteroids, but the reason for this is not clear.

Equine Infectious Anemia

EIA virus is another retrovirus in the lentivirus group. Infection with EIA virus is discussed in more detail in Chapter 18 since the anemia is usually hemolytic. Some horses, however, have anemia that appears to be nonregenerative. Differentiation is difficult because reticulocytes rarely circulate in horses.

Rickettsial Infections and Hemobartonelloses

Anemia commonly is present in dogs with ehrlichiosis and is usually nonregenerative unless it is caused by hemorrhage from thrombocytopenia, or if hemolysis from concurrent babesiosis is present. The marrow may be hypercellular with an increased M/E ratio in the acute phase, but the chronic phase is characterized by pancytopenia and hypoplasia of the marrow except for plasmacytosis, which is regularly present. Most canine ehrlichiosis in the United States is caused by *Ehrlichia canis*, which infects primarily monocytes. Recently a granulocytic ehrlichiosis was found in dogs in the eastern part of the United States, possibly associated with *Ehrlichia equi* or *E. ewingii*; In New York and New England, the prevalence of both human and canine granulocytic ehrlichiosis may be increasing. Platelets seem to be affected primarily, but a normocytic normochromic anemia and sometimes polyarthritis can occur as well. A common presentation is epistaxis or other mucosal bleeding.

Hemobartonellosis in cats sometimes is associated with nonregenerative anemia. *Haemobartonella felis* recently has been reclassified as a mycoplasma. The organism may be an opportunist, affecting immunosuppressed or debilitated cats. These cats should be tested for retroviruses or other abnormalities. Even if only occasional *Haemobartonella* organisms are seen in a cat with a nonregenerative anemia, the organisms may be contributing to the anemia and the cat should be treated.

Ch26 Drugs, Toxins, and Metabolic Causes of Nonregenerative Anemia

Drugs Causing Nonregenerative Anemia or Pancytopenia

Cancer chemotherapy*

    Alkylating agents – cyclophosphamide, melphalan, busulfan, chlorambucil
    Antibiotics – doxorubicin, mitoxantrone, actinomycin D
    Antimetabolites – methotrexate, cytarabine
    Others – carboplatin, nitrosoureas, hydroxyurea

Estrogen

    Estradiol cyclopentylpropionate (ECP)

Nonsteroidal anti-inflammatory drugs

    Phenylbutazone, meclofenamic acid

Antibacterials

    Sulfonamides, trimethoprim, cefadroxil, chloramphenicol

Anticonvulsants

    Phenobarbitol, primidone, phentoin

Other

    Albendazole, fenbendazole, propylthiouracil, methimazole
    Quinidine, griseofulvin, thiacetasamide

---

*Most cause neutropenia $\pm$ thrombocytopenia rather than anemia

Toxins such as benzene, phenol, organophosphate, and chlorinated hydrocarbon insecticides can suppress all cell lines of the marrow, although the number of reported cases in pets is low. Drugs have been implicated more commonly (**Figure**).

Anticancer drugs including alkylating agents, anthracyclines, and antimetabolites are myelosuppressive. Neutropenia is most likely to occur because the neutrophil life span in the circulation is only a few hours and constant replacement is needed. In more severe cases, platelets may decrease as well, but because of the long life span of circulating red cells (90–120 days), cessation of production for a short time does not cause a significant drop in Hct. Anemia is not a significant problem with most chemotherapeutic drugs. One dog treated with melphalan for 6 months suddenly developed pancytopenia, which improved but did not totally resolve over an additional 6 months after all myelosuppressive drugs were discontinued. Azathioprine, an immune-suppressive drug, has also caused pancytopenia in dogs.

Phenylbutazone, an anti-inflammatory drug that has proved to be safe and effective in horses, has been a significant cause of irreversible aplasia of the marrow in dogs. Pancytopenia and aplastic anemia have developed in dogs given phenylbutazone even at recommended doses used for relatively short periods of time, or after weeks to months. Delayed metabolism or clearance of the drug has been observed in some humans who developed aplastic anemia after treatment, but this has not been investigated in affected dogs. Periodic monitoring of the hemogram is indicated but significant damage to the marrow has already occurred by the time changes are first detectable on the hemogram.

Chloramphenicol causes a dose-dependent marrow suppression, more severe in cats than dogs. The irreversible idiosyncratic marrow aplasia seen in humans has not been reported in dogs or cats. Because aplastic anemia has occurred in humans after minimal exposure, one must consider the risks to pet owners handling oral preparations, and gloves should be worn when the drug is given. Safer antibiotics are available for most canine and feline infections, so chloramphenicol is rarely the antibiotic of choice.

Sulfonamides, especially those containing trimethoprim, act as folate antagonists causing normocytic normochromic anemia without megaloblastosis, and in rare cases, aplastic anemia.

Albendazole and fenbendazole can cause reversible cytopenias in dogs and cats treated for parasites. A dose-dependent marrow suppression had been demonstrated in beagles during drug development.

Anticonvulsants such as phenobarbitol, primidone, and phenytoin can cause neutropenia, thrombocytopenia, or pancytopenia. Methimazole has caused reversible leukopenia and thrombocytopenia in up to 20% of cats treated for hyperthyroidism. Despite this, it has fewer adverse hematological effects than does the previously used propylthiouracil.

Griseofulvin can cause aplastic anemia in cats, especially those infected with retroviruses. Since immunosuppression predisposes to ringworm infection, these cats are also the most likely to receive the drug. Alternative treatments should be used if possible.

The mechanisms of marrow damage from drugs may be direct toxicity to progenitors, immune-mediated destruction, or interference with enzymes or other hematopoietic factors. Any animal presenting with red cell aplasia or pancytopenia should be evaluated for exposure to toxins or drugs, and whenever possible these should be eliminated. Depending on the offending agent, recovery may be rapid or the effect may be irreversible.

Bracken fern poisoning in cattle causes pancytopenia and irreversible aplasia of the marrow.

Hyperestrogenism

Elevated estrogen concentration interferes with stem cell differentiation and results in pancytopenia and aplastic anemia. Estrogen concentrations may be increased because of endogenous or iatrogenic causes. The toxic effects of estrogen in dogs are well known and have been studied best in cases of iatrogenic overdose of estrogens, especially estradiol cyclopentylpropionate (ECP), which was used in the past to prevent pregnancy or treat prostatic hyperplasia. Evaluation of sequential hemograms shows that neutrophilia occurs in the first 2–3 weeks, followed by neutropenia, thrombocytopenia, and anemia. The dogs that recover do so after 1–2 months; however, most affected dogs die.

Hyperestrogenism and pancytopenia have been seen in male dogs with Sertoli cell and other testicular tumors, and rarely in female dogs with granulosa cell tumors of the ovary. Most male dogs show signs of feminization, and in most of them the involved testicle is abdominal. Surgical removal of the tumor is necessary for any chance of recovery, but the complication rate is high. Affected dogs are at high risk of infections and hemorrhage secondary to neutropenia and thrombocytopenia.

An estrogen-induced, often fatal pancytopenia occurs related to the estrous cycle of female ferrets. They may remain in nearly a constant state of estrus in spring and summer if ovulation is not induced. For this reason, ovariohysterectomy should be performed on all young female pet ferrets that are not to be bred.

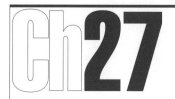

Bone Marrow Failure

Examination of Marrow

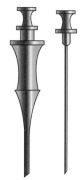

Bone marrow aspiration
needle with stylet

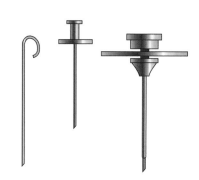

Bone marrow biopsy needle with
stylet and decise to push biopsy
out of the needle

	Aspration	Biopsy
Technique	1-2 drops of marrow smeared on slide and stained	Tissue sample core fixed and stained like other tissue biopsies
Advantages	Best to examine morphology and identify individual cells	Best to assess degree of cellularity and presence of fibrosis or fat infiltration (aplastic anemia)
	Cytologic evaluation	Histologic evaluation

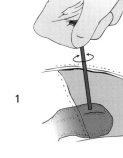

1

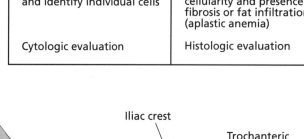

Iliac crest

Trochanteric
fossa

Head of
humerus

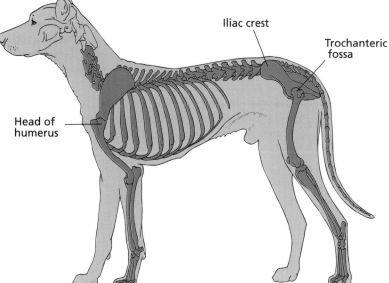

Sites for performing bone marrow aspiration or biopsy

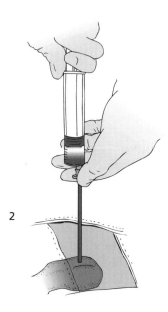

2

Aspiration technique: (1) Advance aspiration needle
with alternating/rotating motion and steady pressure.
(2) Remove stylet and attach syringe.
(3)Aspirate marrow sample

When the hematopoietic cells of the marrow are suppressed or destroyed, the patient develops pancytopenia. Whenever pancytopenia is seen on a hemogram and the cause is not known, the marrow is examined to determine the cause and to try to determine if the damage is reversible. Both aspirates and core biopsy specimens are examined (**Figure**). *See* Chapter 20.

Causes of pancytopenia include stem cell failure, toxic or ischemic marrow damage, abnormal development, and malignant infiltration.

Aplastic Anemia

The number of pluripotent stem cells in the marrow is fixed at birth, and as stem cells are lost, they are not replaced. When the number of stem cells drops below a critical level needed for self-renewal, the marrow becomes depleted and the marrow cavity fills with fat. This progressive atrophy is referred to as *aplastic anemia*. Even though the term mentions only anemia, pancytopenia is seen in the blood.

Most cases of aplastic anemia are idiopathic. In humans a correctable cause is identified in <10% of patients, but some physical, chemical, infectious, and immune-mediated causes are recognized. Ionizing radiation at doses >7 Gy will cause permanent aplasia of the marrow. Some cases in humans, dogs, and perhaps cats appear to be immune mediated, with antibodies directed against stem cells or growth factors.

A syndrome of reversible aplastic anemia was observed at Tufts University in 7 dogs <2 years old. In these dogs, the marrow recovered in as short a time as 2–3 weeks or as long as 4–5 months after diagnosis. An immune-mediated or possibly a viral cause was suspected but not proved.

In cats, FeLV can cause suppression of any or all cell lines and is probably the most common cause of aplastic anemia. In humans, viruses such as hepatitis virus, herpes (Epstein-Barr) virus, or parvovirus (B19) have been implicated as causes of red cell aplasia or aplastic anemia. Feline parvovirus (panleukopenia) causes in vitro inhibition of both granulocytic and erythroid progenitor cells. Since the disease is so acute, anemia generally is not seen clinically.

Marrow Stromal Disorders

Myelofibrosis is probably a manifestation of end-stage marrow failure. In humans, there is cytogenetic evidence that a specific syndrome of myelofibrosis with myeloid metaplasia of the spleen and liver is associated with a clonal (malignant) expansion of granulocyte precursors and a reactive (nonmalignant) proliferation of fibroblasts. Excessive platelet-derived growth factor has been implicated in the stimulation of fibroblasts. Eventually pancytopenia develops as fibrosis fills the marrow. How myelofibrosis in dogs and cats fits into this picture is not known. Probably it is secondary to chronic marrow suppression or damage, for example, by FeLV infection of cats.

During fetal development, the liver and later the spleen are sites of hematopoiesis, and these organs may revert to their previous role in situations such as myelofibrosis or dysplasia. This phenomenon is referred to as *myeloid metaplasia* or *extramedullary hematopoiesis* (EMH). Unfortunately the spleen is not an efficient producer of hematopoietic cells, and EMH is seldom of any benefit in producing adequate numbers of hematopoietic cells. In fact, it may even be detrimental in that the very large spleen may remove more blood cells than it produces through the mechanism of hypersplenism.

Marrow necrosis is rare, and may be secondary to thrombosis or circulatory failure in animals with sepsis, endotoxemia, drug toxicity, malignancy, or viral infection. Pancytopenia is seen only in severe diffuse cases.

Osteosclerosis, which can be observed radiographically as increased bone density, has been reported rarely as an end-stage, irreversible change in chronic marrow abnormalities such as pyruvate kinase deficiency in the dog or FeLV infection in the cat.

Myelodysplasia occurs most frequently in cats, often in association with FeLV infection. The spectrum of the disease ranges from chronic nonregenerative anemia, sometimes with other cytopenias, to a "preleukemic" state with gradually increasing numbers of blasts in the marrow until acute leukemia eventually occurs. *See* Chapter 54. Myelodysplasia has a cellular marrow, which helps to distinguish it from aplastic anemia or myelofibrosis. The reason for the disparity is that hematopoiesis is ineffective, and many abnormal cells die while still in the marrow. Iron stores are increased in the marrow as a result of intramedullary loss of erythroid precursors. The red cells may be macrocytic but without reticulocytosis.

Examination of the Bone Marrow

Indications for examination of marrow include nonregenerative anemia, unexplained thrombocytopenia, neutropenia, and suspected hematopoietic neoplasia.

The M/E ratio allows a rough comparison of granulocyte and monocyte production with erythroid production and should be in the range of 1:1. In both cell lines, only a few blasts and immature precursors should be present. The number of cells increases with progression toward maturation. The M/E ratio may be decreased after severe recent hemorrhage or hemolysis or increased with severe inflammation or nonregenerative anemia. Increased megakaryocyte numbers may be seen when platelets are being destroyed or consumed. Decreased megakaryocyte numbers may be seen in marrow failure or infiltration. The morphology of the cells as well as the presence of any abnormal cells is noted.

A   **Reasons for Increased Hematocrits**

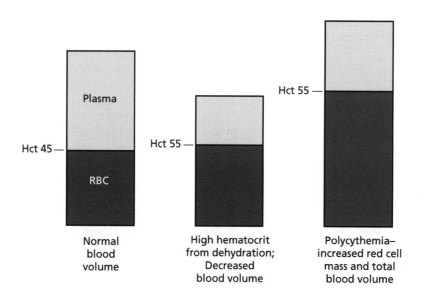

B   **Causes of Polycythemia**

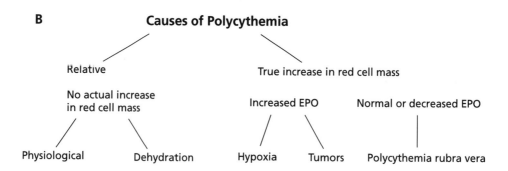

Polycythemia is characterized by the presence of too many red cells in the circulation. It is important to distinguish between true polycythemia and a high Hct. The Hct refers only to the percentage of the blood volume made up of red cells. When excited, a normal animal might have a transient mild increase in Hct because epinephrine causes splenic contraction and a release of additional red cells to the circulation. Normal greyhounds have a Hct of 55%–65%.

Polycythemia may be relative, with an increase in Hct secondary to a decreased plasma volume, not associated with an increased total red cell mass (**Part A**). Absolute polycythemia may occur secondary to increased production of erythropoietin or to an autonomous overproduction of red cells (polycythemia rubra vera) caused by a malignant stem cell disorder.

Regardless of the cause of the increased Hct, the red cell count per microliter and the hemoglobin concentration will increase proportionally at the same time.

Relative Polycythemia Caused by Dehydration

Probably the most common cause of an elevated Hct in veterinary patients is dehydration with loss of plasma volume. The fact that a patient is dehydrated is usually evident in the history or physical examination. Vomiting or diarrhea with inadequate fluid replacement are common causes of dehydration. Clinical signs include dry mouth, sunken eyes, and loss of cutaneous elasticity. Particularly in dogs and cats, if the skin over the back is lifted, it may remain that way instead of immediately falling back into place. The extent of dehydration often can be estimated by the severity of these signs. If the fluid loss is rapid, the only signs might be a deep-red color and dryness of the oral mucous membranes. Assuming that the plasma proteins are otherwise normal, dehydration is characterized by an elevation of the total serum protein concentration, including albumin and globulin, in addition to an increased Hct. The increase in albumin is especially significant because no known disease causes an actual increase in albumin; thus, any increase is caused by a loss of fluid. A combination of these clinical and laboratory findings usually makes diagnosis of dehydration relatively simple. Correction of the problem is achieved by appropriate fluid replacement.

Polycythemia Secondary to Increased Erythropoietin

Erythropoietin may be increased for 1 of 2 reasons: as a response to hypoxia or because of oversecretion from a population of malignant cells, usually in the kidney. In a normal animal, erythropoietin secretion is regulated by the amount of oxygen in the blood perfusing the kidneys. Whenever atmospheric oxygen tension is low, for example, at high altitudes, erythropoietin secretion increases and within a few days, the Hct rises to provide more red cells to deliver oxygen.

Patients with chronic lung disease might experience hypoxia and have an elevated Hct. With some types of heart disease, especially those associated with a right-to-left shunting of blood (e.g., tetralogy of Fallot), a mixture of oxygenated and unoxygenated blood will go to the peripheral circulation including the kidneys. Rarely, chronic abnormalities in the ability of hemoglobin to carry or deliver oxygen occur. An example might be elevated methemoglobin due to a congenital deficiency of methemoglobin reductase.

Erythropoietin may be secreted autonomously by certain kinds of tumors. This has been seen most commonly in dogs with renal adenocarcinoma or renal lymphoma. Rarely, tumors in other sites cause polycythemia. Examples include hepatic and nasal tumors of dogs. In humans, other renal abnormalities such as cysts or vascular abnormalities have caused polycythemia. The cause in these latter cases is more likely interference with circulation and oxygen delivery to the kidney, rather than autonomous overproduction of erythropoietin.

Polycythemia Rubra Vera

In polycythemia rubra vera, a malignant clone of red cells proliferates despite normal or low concentrations of erythropoietin. The red cells produced function normally, but too many are produced. It is the red cell equivalent of chronic lymphocytic or myelogenous leukemia. Splenomegaly is usually present, and sometimes white cell and platelet counts are increased. This is discussed in more detail in Chapter 55.

Manifestations of Polycythemia

Polycythemia of any cause causes clinical signs by increasing the volume and viscosity of blood (**Part B**). When this happens, the mucous membranes become red, the blood pressure rises, and signs of mental dullness and dyspnea from decreased cerebral perfusion and heart failure can occur.

Once it is determined that dehydration can be ruled out as a cause of an increased Hct, the heart and lungs are evaluated by physical examination, radiography, measurement of the oxygen content of the blood, and other specific tests of heart or lung function. In general, the signs of the underlying heart or lung disease are severe and chronic before the Hct begins to rise, and the source of the problem is evident. If cardiac and pulmonary diseases can be ruled out, then the kidneys are evaluated, usually by ultrasonography, which should show the presence or absence of a renal mass.

Erythropoietin concentrations increase when hypoxia of any cause is present. In polycythemia rubra vera, the concentrations are typically normal or low, since the malignant clone of erythroid cells continues to proliferate independently of erythropoietin secretion.

Evaluation of the bone marrow is less likely to help with a diagnosis because increased erythroid production is present regardless of the cause. Sometimes polycythemia rubra vera may be associated with abnormalities in the granulocytic or megakaryocytic cell lines.

Ch 29 Evaluation

A   Quantitative Buffy Coat (QBC)

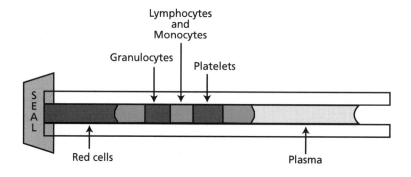

Differentiated cell layers in centrifuged QBC blood tube used
to estimate numbers of red cells, each type of white cell and platelets.

B   Description of an Abnormal Canine Hemogram

	Percentage	Total WBC Count	Reference Range
WBC	100%	20,000/μL	6,000 – 17,000
Neutrophils	88%	17,600/μL	3,000 – 11,000
Lymphocytes	4%	800/μL	1,000 – 5,000
Monocytes	8%	1,600/μL	0 – 1,500
Eosinophils	0%	0/μL	0 – 1,000

This hemogram portrays a neutrophilic leukocytosis with lymphopenia,
monocytosis. and eosinopenia.

    The WBC is above the limits of the reference range (leukocytosis).
The neutrophil (neutrophilia) and monocyte (monocytosis) counts are
increased and the lymphocyte (lymphopenia) and eosinophil (eosinopenia)
counts are decreased.

WBC Count, Expressed as 10^6 Cells/µL

The evaluation of the number and types of WBCs is an important part of CBC.

The WBC (leukocyte) count can be performed either manually or semiautomatically. A hemocytometer WBC count compares favorably with an electronically determined WBC count (5%–10% variation), but semiautomated counts are used routinely by most veterinary laboratories. Red cells are hemolyzed so they will not interfere with the counting of white cells. Otherwise the count is performed in a manner similar to that used for red cells. Any nucleated red cells are counted as white cells, and a correction is made later.

In the flow cytometric method, individual cells are made to traverse a flow-through cell detector in single file through the path of a focused laser beam. The cells scatter the light at different angles depending on cell size, nuclear complexity, internal granularity, and surface morphology.

Becton Dickinson QBC (Quantitative Buffy Coat)

The QBC centrifugal hematology system utilizes cell staining and density-gradient centrifugation to determine white cell and platelet counts (in addition to Hct) by means of a modified microhematocrit procedure (**Part A**). In the QBC method, cells in the buffy coat are stained by a reagent, and the resulting packed cell layers are mechanically expanded during high-speed centrifugation and the lengths of the differentiated cell layers are then measured. Hct, platelet count, total WBC count, and estimated counts of the granulocyte and lymphocyte/monocyte subpopulations can be determined. Evaluation of a stained blood smear should still be done to look for morphological abnormalities.

Differential WBC Count, Expressed as 10^3 Cells/µL or %

The differential count is performed by examining a stained blood smear with an oil immersion objective and classifying each of 100 nucleated cells according to its type (e.g., neutrophil, lymphocyte). The differential count expressed as a percentage indicates the number of each type relative to the total (e.g., 72% neutrophils, 18% lymphocytes). The absolute number of a particular cell type is calculated by multiplying the total WBC count by the percentage for each type. *The absolute numbers should be used in interpreting leukocyte patterns.* The differential count, expressed as 10^3 cells/µL (e.g., 8,592 neutrophils, 2,148 lymphocytes), indicates the absolute number of each cell type per microliter of blood.

Because nucleated red cells are counted as white cells by either electronic or manual counting methods, the raw WBC count must be corrected for the presence of nucleated red cells. This is done by keeping a separate count of the number of nucleated red cells counted during the counting of 100 WBCs. The correction is 100/(100 + number of nucleated red cells) × uncorrected WBC count. For example, if 9 nucleated red cells were counted in addition to the 100 WBCs, then only 100/109 of the total WBC count per microliter would really be WBCs. This correction must be made before the absolute number of each type of WBC is determined.

Depending on total and differential cell counts, the leukogram is described and interpreted. The term *leukocytosis* is used to describe a leukocyte count greater than the upper limit of the reference range for the species in question. One also should mention increases in specific cells: neutrophilia, lymphocytosis, monocytosis, eosinophilia, or basophilia. Increases can be absolute (number of cells/µL) or relative (percentage of total WBC count); *common usage refers to absolute numbers* not relative numbers. A leukocyte count below the lower limit of the reference range for the given species is called *leukopenia*. The terms for decreases in specific cells are e.g., neutropenia, lymphopenia, eosinopenia. The presence of bands in numbers >100–300/µL, or the presence of less mature cells of the neutrophilic series (metamyelocytes, myelocytes, promyelocytes, or myeloblasts) in the circulation also should be noted. The left shift is "degenerative" if the number of bands exceeds the number of segmented neutrophils. The example in **Part B** illustrates the *description* of an abnormal canine leukogram.

Additional terms may be used to describe morphologic changes (toxic changes) in neutrophils that might be associated with inflammation or tissue damage. These toxic changes include toxic granules, small to medium-sized vacuoles, and basophilic cytoplasm. The nucleus may be hypersegmented with loose, swollen-appearing chromatin. Döhle bodies are small (1–2 µ), round or oval, gray-blue bodies in the cytoplasm of neutrophils. They are derived from incomplete utilization of RNA during maturation of the cytoplasm.

In addition to morphologic changes in neutrophils, lymphocytes may be described as "reactive," indicating a response to an antigen. A reactive lymphocyte contains dark-blue cytoplasm and a nuclear chromatin that is somewhat less condensed than that of a small lymphocyte.

Interpretation of the Leukogram

After the numbers of various types of WBCs have been determined and any changes described, the changes must be interpreted. Leukocyte patterns in peripheral blood reflect a balance between the production and release of cells from the marrow, their distribution in blood vessels, their life span, migration from vessels into tissue, and the rate of destruction. Various disease processes may elicit changes in the leukogram that vary with the intensity and duration of the disease process as well as with the cause, the virulence of an infectious agent, the species of patient, individual hematopoietic reactivity, location of the process, and therapy. Increases in white cell counts may be physiologic or pathologic and decreases are always pathologic.

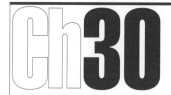

Granulopoiesis (Neutrophil Production)

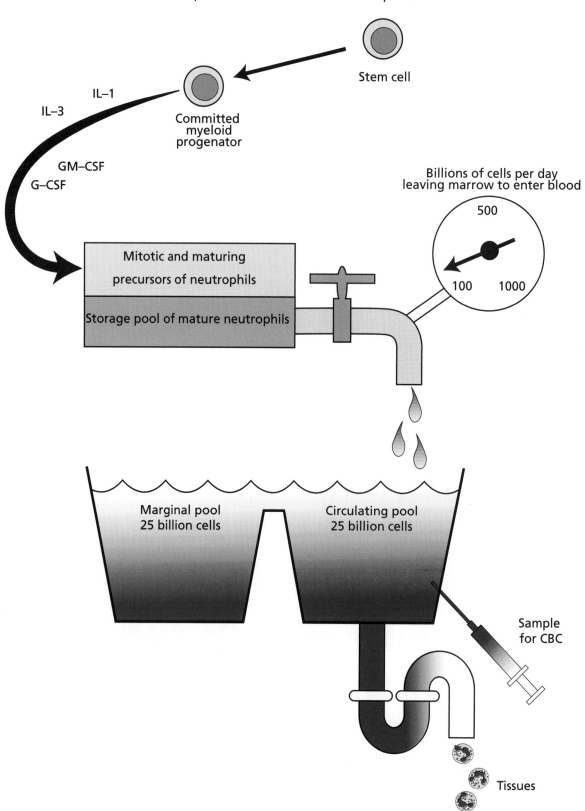

Granulopoiesis and "Pools" of Neutrophils

Stem cell

IL–1
IL–3
Committed myeloid progenator

GM–CSF
G–CSF

Billions of cells per day leaving marrow to enter blood

500
100   1000

Mitotic and maturing precursors of neutrophils

Storage pool of mature neutrophils

Marginal pool 25 billion cells

Circulating pool 25 billion cells

Sample for CBC

Tissues

The events of early hematopoiesis were described in Chapter 2. Pluripotent stem cells under the direction of growth factors give rise to committed progenitors. The progenitors destined to become neutrophils or monocytes respond initially to the same growth signals and factors, especially IL-3 and GM-CSF. Control of eosinophils and basophils is separate.

Production of Neutrophils in the Marrow

The mitotic pool consists of the myeloblast, which has a round nucleus and a visible nucleolus. The promyelocyte (progranulocyte) is slightly larger than the myeloblast and contains azurophilic "primary" granules in the cytoplasm. The primary granules are membrane-bound lysosomes containing a number of enzymes and other factors. Many granules visible at this stage are not as clearly seen in later stages. Primary granules are split among daughter cells during later mitotic divisions and also undergo metabolic changes, which decrease their stainability with Wright's stain. The most mature cell that is still capable of mitosis is the myelocyte, which is slightly smaller than the myeloblast. The nucleus is still round, secondary granules appear, and primary granules are sparse. Secondary granules (lysosomes) contain lysosomal and other bacteriostatic substances.

The neutrophilic myelocyte and its progeny have prominent granules in some species such as humans, whereas those of most domestic animal species are invisible or very faint. Some species such as rabbits, guinea pigs, birds, and reptiles have both primary (blue) and secondary (pink) granules visible; in those species the cells are called *heterophils* instead of neutrophils.

Cells in the maturation pool can no longer divide, but in the normal animal, continue to mature in the marrow (**Figure**). The earliest of these cells is the metamyelocyte. The nucleus is indented and chromatin is more consolidated. As the nucleus continues to indent, it takes the shape of a U or an S, and is then called a *band neutrophil*. The sides of the nucleus are approximately uniform in diameter throughout its length without any indentations or kinks. Mature neutrophils have a nucleus with 3–5 lobes connected by a thin filament of chromatin in humans, but the lobes are frequently difficult to see in neutrophils of domestic animals.

The morphological distinction between mature neutrophils and band neutrophils is arbitrary and what any one cell is called may vary from one person to another. Normally the band neutrophil should have the membranes parallel all around the nucleus. As soon as an indentation occurs, the cell becomes a mature neutrophil. The cytoplasm in dog, cat, and horse neutrophils is normally clear to light gray. The cytoplasm in cattle and some primate neutrophils (including humans) may stain a pale-pink color that sometimes is mistaken for eosinophil granules. Neutrophils have several names that are synonymous: polymorphonuclear leukocyte, poly, segmented neutrophil, and seg.

The time required for development of a mature neutrophil varies to some extent between species, but generally ranges from 2 to 7 days. The total generation time (blast to mature neutrophil) may be shortened, and some divisions may be skipped when increased need for neutrophils is present. In the dog, progression from myelocyte to neutrophil under the stimulation of G-CSF requires about 2–3 days. This can be an advantage if the need for neutrophils is acute and severe, since it is not necessary to begin at the myeloblast stage whenever new neutrophils are needed.

Some mature neutrophils remain in the storage pool of marrow after maturation is complete. The storage pool is very large in some species. In the dog, the storage pool contains up to a 5-day supply of mature neutrophils, but in ruminants the storage pool is much smaller. There are some important clinical implications of these species differences. The release of neutrophils from the marrow is aged-ordered. During periods of increased demand for neutrophils, the storage pool of mature cells is depleted before a significant number of band neutrophils are released into the blood.

Neutrophils in the Blood

Circulating neutrophils are on their way to the tissues where they function to protect against invasion, primarily by bacteria. Within the vasculature at any one time, about half of the neutrophils are in the circulating pool, in which neutrophils move with the blood flow (see **Figure**). This is the pool of cells sampled by blood collection. The other half are in the marginated pool, with cells settled along vessel walls, mostly in capillaries and venules. Neutrophils move freely back and forth between the 2 pools. Whenever neutrophils are needed in the tissues, neutrophils in the marginated pool are the first to move out of the circulation. The circulating half-life of a neutrophil is about 6–10 hours (average life span, 8–12 hours). Thus, all circulating neutrophils are replaced 2–3 times daily. Once neutrophils leave the circulation, they never return.

Some species variation in the number of circulating neutrophils and lymphocytes exists. For example, horses have relatively equal numbers of neutrophils and lymphocytes, dogs and cats have more neutrophils than lymphocytes, and the opposite is true for ruminants. In ruminants, the neutrophil-lymphocyte ratio increases in the presence of inflammation.

A   Anatomy of the Mature Neutrophil

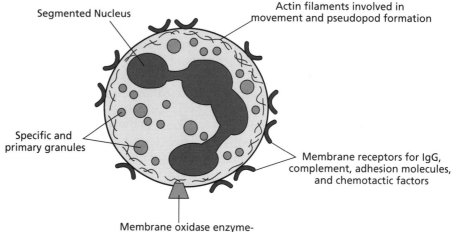

Segmented Nucleus

Actin filaments involved in movement and pseudopod formation

Specific and primary granules

Membrane receptors for IgG, complement, adhesion molecules, and chemotactic factors

Membrane oxidase enzyme- when stimulated converts oxygen to superoxide ion (O_2^-) and hydrogen peroxide (H_2O_2)

B   The Life of a Neutrophil

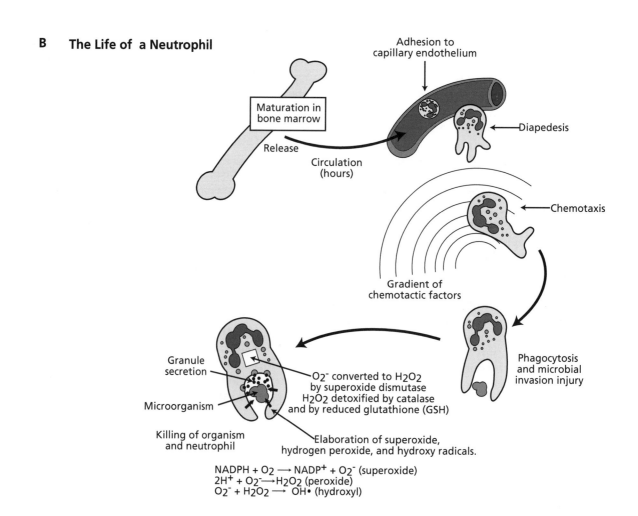

Adhesion to capillary endothelium

Maturation in bone marrow

Release

Diapedesis

Circulation (hours)

Chemotaxis

Gradient of chemotactic factors

Phagocytosis and microbial invasion injury

Granule secretion

O_2^- converted to H_2O_2 by superoxide dismutase H_2O_2 detoxified by catalase and by reduced glutathione (GSH)

Microorganism

Killing of organism and neutrophil

Elaboration of superoxide, hydrogen peroxide, and hydroxy radicals.

$$NADPH + O_2 \longrightarrow NADP^+ + O_2^- \text{ (superoxide)}$$
$$2H^+ + O_2^- \longrightarrow H_2O_2 \text{ (peroxide)}$$
$$O_2^- + H_2O_2 \longrightarrow OH\bullet \text{ (hydroxyl)}$$

As neutrophils mature in the marrow, they change their appearance and develop biochemical and functional characteristics that allow them to move in an organized manner, to phagocytize particulate matter, and to kill ingested microorganisms.

The nucleus is nonfunctional and contains several lobes. The cytoplasm contains primary and secondary (specific) granules. These granules contain highly active toxic oxygen metabolites, which when released from the granules will kill bacteria and the neutrophil itself. A fibrous network made up primarily of actin is located beneath the plasma membrane. The actin reacts with myosin, just as it does in muscle cells, and allows the neutrophil to move in an ameboid manner. The source of energy for this motion is glycolysis.

The surface of the neutrophil contains (**Part A**) adhesion molecules, which interact with receptors on the endothelium to allow the neutrophil to adhere and to exit the circulation (diapedesis) to the tissues. *See* Chapter 41. The external membrane of the neutrophil contains receptors for IgG and complement. Neutrophils "recognize" foreign material when it becomes coated (opsonized, which comes from the Greek word meaning "prepared for dining") by complement or antibody. The neutrophil has a special advantage in attaching to opsinized bacteria prior to phagocytosis. Neutrophils can phagocytize bacteria in the absence of immunoglobulin, but somewhat less efficiently.

Chemotaxis

Neutrophils respond to a stimulus along a chemical gradient. The response requires proper recognition of the stimulant and a functional cytoskeleton for motility. Examples of chemotactic factors include endotoxin produced by certain gram-negative bacteria, antigen-antibody complexes, substances released from granules of other neutrophils, bacterial peptides, denatured proteins, coagulation factors, and complement.

Ingestion/Endocytosis

The cell membrane of the neutrophil invaginates (or folds in) and then surrounds the foreign material (see **Part B**). A vacuole (phagosome) containing the ingested material then forms. Lysosomes, granules containing digestive substances, combine with the phagosomes to form a phagolysosome. The contents of the lysosome are released into the cytoplasm of the neutrophil and may leak into the surrounding tissue. The presence of these lysosomal substances in the tissues will enhance and perpetuate inflammation by damaging normal tissues and by attracting additional neutrophils. Lysosomes also contain substances that cause fever (pyrogens).

Oxygen-Dependent Microbial Killing

As the contents of the granules are secreted into the forming phagolysosome, the membrane generates toxic oxygen metabolites such as superoxide anion and hydrogen peroxide (H_2O_2) and hydroxyl radicals. The microorganism is exposed to these as it is being enveloped by pseudopods extended by the membrane of the neutrophil. The mechanism by which active oxygen metabolites are formed (respiratory burst) is shown in **Part B**.

At the same time, the enzyme myeloperoxidase (MPO), found in primary granules, works with H_2O_2 and a halide such as chloride to form a potent antimicrobial system effective against bacteria, fungi, viruses, mycoplasma, sperm, and tumor cells: $MPO + H_2O_2 + Cl^- \rightarrow HOCl$ (hypochlorous acid, the same compound found in bleach).

Oxygen-Independent Microbial Killing

An acid pH results from the by-products of inflammation and enhances the activity of some lysosomal enzymes. Lysozyme generated in neutrophil granules is capable of hydrolyzing the cell wall of a few bacteria by exposure to antibody, complement, or hydrogen peroxide.

Lactoferrin is found in milk and many other secretions and exudates. It binds iron and acts to inhibit bacterial growth. This may partially explain the finding of low serum iron levels in inflammatory and chronic diseases.

Control of Bactericidal Products

The neutrophil has several mechanisms to protect it and surrounding tissues against bystander damage from the antimicrobial substances. Superoxide dismutase protects against oxidation of cell proteins by the superoxide radical. Catalase and reduced glutathione destroy excess hydrogen peroxide. The same effect of glutathione serves to protect red cells against oxidant toxin. Ascorbate and vitamin E function as antioxidants.

Neutrophil Function Disorders

Neutrophils may be affected adversely by outside effects like a corticosteroid-mediated decrease in chemotaxis and have inherited abnormalities.

If neutrophils are unable to adhere to the endothelial surface, they will be unable to leave the circulation to function in the tissues. Adhesion defects have been described in humans, cattle (known as bovine leukocyte adhesion defect, BLAD), and dogs. It is a recessive trait in which the carriers are normal. The disease is characterized by recurring bacterial infections with severe neutrophilia and a lack of pus formation at the site of the infection. A defect in the hexose monophosphate shunt in neutrophils causes a reduced ability to kill bacteria, a rare autosomal recessive trait reported in Irish Setters.

The Pelger-Huët Anomaly found in dogs and cats, is characterized by hyposegmentation of the nucleus of neutrophils usually with no clinical signs.

Chédiak-Higashi Syndrome is a defect in microtubules resulting in large abnormal granule formation in leukocytes and melanocytes, and some abnormality in neutrophil motility. Affected animals have silver-gray hair.

Ch32 Patterns of Change in Neutrophil Numbers

A. Mechanisms of Neutrophilia

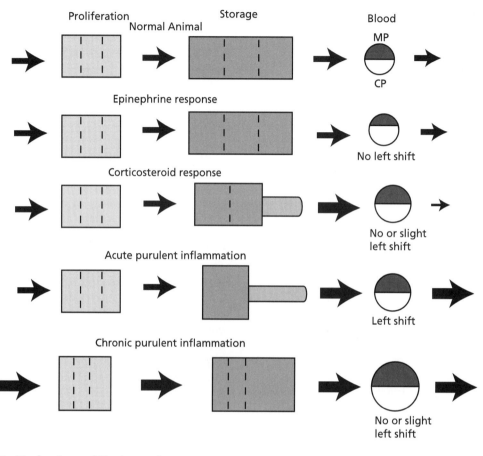

B. Mechanisms of Neutropenia

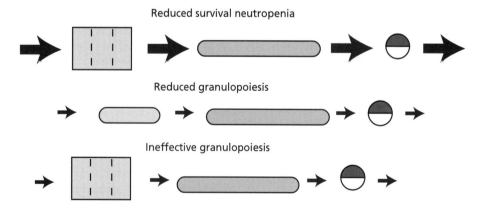

Size of arrows represent rates of movement of cells through the compartments of granulopoiesis, marrow storage, and blood. The size of the tubes, circle, and shaded area represent bone marrow proliferation and storage pools, blood circulating (CP), and marginated (MP) neutrophil pools, respectively.

Leukocytosis and Neutrophilia

Physiologic Leukocytosis (Epinephrine Response)

A neutrophilic leukocytosis with as much as a 1–2-fold increase in WBC count and normal to increased numbers of lymphocytes can be observed in healthy young cats, horses, and cattle subjected to exertion or emotional stress. Dogs show such a response less frequently than other species. The response may be noted immediately and is caused by endogenous release of epinephrine, resulting in increased blood pressure and flow velocity. The mechanism of the change is a temporary redistribution of neutrophils within the vascular space (**Part A**), so that the circulating granulocyte pool is increased at the expense of the marginated pool. The effect subsides within a few minutes after the stress is relieved.

Glucocorticoid-Mediated Leukocytosis

Endogenous release or exogenous administration of glucocorticoids causes a release of mature neutrophils from the marrow storage pool. Corticosteroids also inhibit egress of neutrophils into the tissues. At the same time, lymphocytes and eosinophils are sequestered or lysed, depending on the species. A neutrophilic leukocytosis and eosinopenia, lymphopenia, and (in some species) monocytosis result. The neutrophilia may be documented 2–6 hours following stress or steroid therapy.

Inflammation

The neutrophil count reflects a balance between peripheral demand for cells and the rate of production and release of cells from the bone marrow. The most typical response to inflammation is neutrophilia, the magnitude of which depends on the species; the location, severity, and duration of the inflammatory process; and the etiology or etiologic agent. In very acute or overwhelming inflammation, the consumption of neutrophils exceeds the rate of replacement. Thus, inflammation can be associated with neutrophilia, neutropenia, or even a normal neutrophil count. In order to label a leukogram as inflammation, *left shift* (the presence in peripheral blood of band and other immature neutrophils) must be present. The term is derived from the convention of representing the maturation sequence of blood cells with the least mature cell of the series (e.g., myeloblast) at the left and the most mature cell (e.g., segmented neutrophil) at the right.

Degenerative indicates that immature forms outnumber segmented neutrophils. A degenerative left shift is commonly associated with a normal or decreased WBC count, though occasionally the leukocyte count is elevated. The presence of a degenerative left shift signifies an inability of the marrow to meet the peripheral demand for neutrophils. This pattern is usually seen in the early stage of acute, severe inflammation when insufficient time has elapsed for the bone marrow to increase the rate of granulopoiesis. Cattle are the species that most commonly shows inflammation with a degenerative left shift, owing to their smaller marrow reserve of segmented neu-

trophils. In most other species, this pattern may be associated with overwhelming inflammation or endotoxemia when granulopoiesis is inhibited and maturation is suppressed. A persistent degenerative left shift suggests a poor prognosis.

Glucocorticoid stress may accompany inflammation so that lymphopenia and eosinopenia may be present along with left shift.

Neutropenia

Like changes in red cells or platelets, neutropenia can be caused by excessive losses or decreased production (**Part B**). Neutrophils permanently leave the circulation when they are drawn to a site of inflammation. An abrupt drop in circulating neutrophils occurs in the presence of tumor necrosis factor or endotoxin. Whenever neutrophils are consumed more rapidly than they can be replaced, neutropenia is the result. Survival time for neutrophils in the tissues varies from a few days in a normal animal to a few minutes in the presence of severe inflammation.

Decreased production of neutrophils by the bone marrow also results in neutropenia, either by itself or commonly with decreased production of red cells, platelets, or both (aplastic anemia). Whenever hematopoiesis is suppressed for any reason, neutrophils are the first marrow cell line to decrease because of the normally short half-life of the neutrophil in the circulation (6–12 hours). Platelets are the next to decrease in number, and red cell numbers decline slowly because old cells persist over several weeks.

Causes of decreased production of neutrophils include primary bone marrow failure or infiltration with fibrous connective tissue or malignant cells. Some drugs and toxins are known to suppress the marrow. Myelosuppressive anticancer drugs are a common transient cause of severe neutropenia in dogs and cats. With most of these drugs, the lowest count (nadir) occurs about 1 week after the drug is given and rebounds 2–3 days later. Infectious diseases that might cause neutropenia are parvoviruses, retroviruses, and rickettsial diseases.

Some decrease in circulating neutrophils may occur without increasing susceptibility to infections, as a surplus normally is present. In most species, a neutrophil count <1,000/μL is likely to result in infection, often within days after the count drops. Infections are usually bacterial, especially those residing in the intestinal or respiratory tract, with gram-negative enteric flora being the most common.

In animals presenting with sepsis and neutropenia, it may be difficult to differentiate whether the neutropenia is the primary problem or secondary to the sepsis. If neutropenia is secondary to sepsis, the count usually begins to rise as the infection is treated.

A rare inherited disease, cyclic hematopoiesis (gray collie syndrome), may cause neutropenia along with other cytopenias recurring at set intervals. The other cytopenias may be less evident because of longer circulating times. This disease is fatal either because of overwhelming infections or because of systemic amyloidosis.

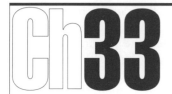

Monocytes and Macrophages

Development and Maturation of Mononuclear Phagocytes

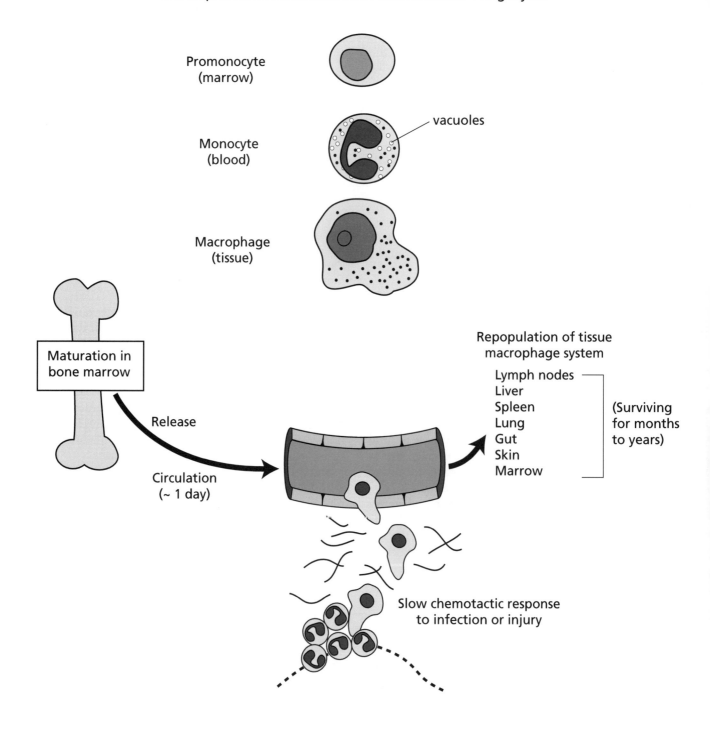

Promonocyte
(marrow)

Monocyte
(blood)

vacuoles

Macrophage
(tissue)

Maturation in
bone marrow

Release

Circulation
(~ 1 day)

Repopulation of tissue
macrophage system

Lymph nodes
Liver
Spleen
Lung
Gut
Skin
Marrow

(Surviving
for months
to years)

Slow chemotactic response
to infection or injury

onocytes arise from a progenitor that also produces neutrophils. IL-3 and GM-CSF regulate the process. Further differentiation to the mature monocyte requires M-CSF, produced by activated monocytes, macrophages, T lymphocytes, and endothelial cells in response to many of the same stimuli that cause neutrophils to be produced.

Maturation from monoblast to promonocyte to monocyte is continuous and takes place more quickly than the maturation of a neutrophil. The mature monocytes are not stored to any extent in the marrow, but enter the circulation as soon as they are mature, so very few immature monocytes are seen in aspirates of bone marrow. For the same reason, when a patient is recovering from a reversible suppression as from drugs or infection of the marrow, monocytosis precedes the return of neutrophils by 1 or 2 days and can be considered as a favorable prognostic sign.

The monocyte is recognizable on smears with Wright's stain as a large cell with a variably shaped nucleus that appears folded or vacuolated. The cytoplasm is gray, sometimes with vacuoles and with an irregular, sometimes poorly defined cell membrane. Sometimes monocytes resemble large lymphocytes.

After 12–26 hours monocytes leave the circulation for various tissues and in contrast to the neutrophil, survive for weeks to years as macrophages (**Figure**). The movement of monocytes out of the circulation is inhibited by corticosteroids. Thus, both neutrophilia and monocytosis may be present in animals treated with steroids. The macrophage, sometimes called a *histiocyte,* is larger than the monocyte, with a round nucleus and prominent nucleolus. The cytoplasm may contain phagocytized material.

Phagocytic Function of Macrophages

Monocytes and macrophages move in the same way to the same chemotactic factors and opsonins as neutrophils. Neutrophils tend to move more quickly and predominate in the first 1 or 2 days of an inflammatory reaction. Monocytes enter organs such as the spleen, lymph nodes, liver, and lungs, where as macrophages they align themselves along blood and lymphatic vessels to filter out microbes and to perform immunological functions. They also trap and remove aged, damaged, or antibody-coated red cells or platelets. Macrophages proliferate in the tissues in response to increased need locally, and even reenter the circulation in some situations. The metabolism of macrophages varies with location. Pulmonary alveolar macrophages have primarily aerobic metabolism, whereas those in hypoxic tissues utilize glycolysis.

Macrophages are more effective than neutrophils in controlling intracellular bacteria such as *Mycobacterium, Listeria,* and *Brucella* species, as well as fungi and protozoa. Ingested organisms are destroyed by oxidative and oxygen-independent mechanisms similar to those of neutrophils. Some protozoal organisms such as *Tox-*

oplasma and *Leishmania* species and viruses such as retroviruses and feline infectious peritonitis (a coronavirus) produce protective substances that allow them to survive in the macrophage.

In addition to removal of microorganisms, macrophages are scavengers of cellular debris and foreign matter. They remove inclusions such as Howell-Jolly bodies, Heinz bodies, or red cell parasites. Mucopolysaccharidosis is a complex of disorders characterized by an accumulation in macrophages of abnormal mucopolysaccharide metabolic by-products.

Sometimes when foreign matter is too large for a single macrophage to ingest, several macrophages surround the substance and fuse to form a multinucleated giant cell. Giant cells may be more numerous in certain granulomatous infections such as tuberculosis.

Immunological and Secretory Functions of Macrophages

A role of macrophages is to recognize and respond to foreign antigens. Macrophages secrete many soluble substances, including IL-1 and TNF, that not only attract lymphocytes, but also cause fever through effects on the hypothalamus and stimulate bone marrow stem cells, platelets, and other procoagulants.

Antigens, in the context of histocompatibility antigens, are presented to helper T cells and B cells on the surface of macrophages. Macrophages determine the amount and form of the antigen to be presented. In turn, lymphocytes produce lymphokines that attract and activate macrophages, which then can nonspecifically destroy organisms. Specialized macrophages, especially Kupffer cells in the liver, can destroy endotoxin absorbed by the intestine.

Macrophages are a major component of the specific and nonspecific immune responses against viral infections. Interferons are released by both macrophages and T cells to block viral replication, and natural killer cells are attracted to lyse virus-infected cells.

Macrophages are important in immune surveillance against malignancy, by recognizing the presence of new tumor-related antigens. Similarly to the detriment of the patient, macrophages can recognize and damage transplanted organs as part of the rejection phenomenon. These responses involve not only macrophages but also lymphocytes, platelets, and neutrophils.

Monocytosis and Monocytopenia

The number of circulating monocytes can increase in any acute or chronic disorder characterized by an increased tissue demand for phagocytes or a cellular immune response. Thus, any process that stimulates neutrophilia would also stimulate monocytosis because of GM-CSF. Monocytosis may occur in response to endogenous or exogenous corticosteroids, especially in the dog.

Because low numbers of circulating monocytes are normally present in the circulation, the absence of monocytes (monocytopenia) is not considered abnormal.

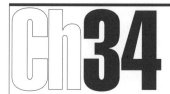

Eosinophils

Appearance and Action of Eosinophils

A

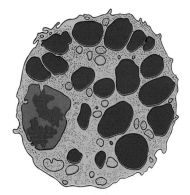

Equine eosinophil (large granules)

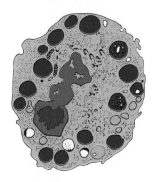

Canine eosinophil

The appearance of eosinophil granules varies between species. The horse eosinophil has much larger granules than those of the dog and other species. Those of the cat (not shown) are rod-shaped rather than round. The red stain of the granules is from abundant quantities of basic protein that has afffinity for acid dyes.

B

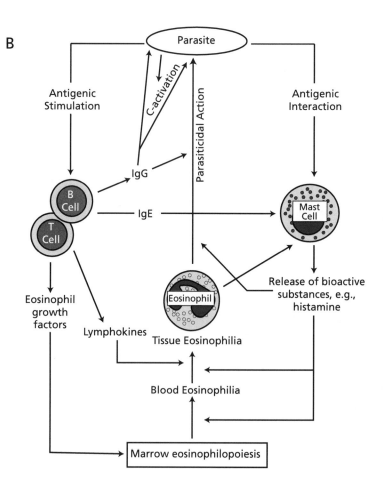

Eosinophils have committed precursor cells that are separate from the CFU-GM, probably a stem cell (CFU-EO), but the maturation sequence is very similar to that of the neutrophil. The hematopoietic growth factors GM-CSF, IL-3, and IL-5 and others increase the production of eosinophils. IL-4 stimulates eosinophil adhesion to the endothelium in preparation for exiting the circulation. Increased numbers of circulating eosinophils (eosinophilia) have been observed in patients treated with IL-2, which stimulates T cells to produce IL-5.

In the marrow, the specific eosinophil granules are first recognizable at the myelocyte stage, allowing eosinophils to be differentiated morphologically from basophil or neutrophil precursors. The granules are large and stain pink to orange with Wright's stain (**Part A**). The contents of the granules, major basic protein, superoxide and peroxidase are especially toxic to helminth and protozoal parasites. Eosinophil granules also contain histaminase and plasminogen.

The eosinophil is slightly larger than a neutrophil and the nuclei are similar, but the degree of segmentation of eosinophil and basophil nuclei may be less than that of the neutrophil. Eosinophils have abilities for diapedesis and chemotaxis similar to those of the neutrophil, but the stimuli are different. Mature eosinophils circulate for only a few hours, then migrate to tissues where they survive several days to as long as several weeks. They do not reenter the circulation once they leave.

Stimulation for production and chemotaxis is mediated by soluble factors produced by sensitized T lymphocytes, macrophages, and mast cells (**Part B**). Some of these factors are immune complexes involving IgE, eosinophil chemotactic factor of anaphylaxis, platelet-activating factor, histamine, activated complement, leukotrienes, and prostaglandins. Eosinophils may play a role in the immune response by acting as antigen-presenting cells. The initial binding of eosinophils to parasites is via IgE and complement opsonization. Although eosinophils have some ability to phagocytize and kill bacteria, they are more adept at killing parasites. Eosinophils inhibit histamine, the primary mediator of immediate type I hypersensitivity, and moderate the edema-producing effects of serotonin and bradykinin. While some products released from activated eosinophils enhance the host defenses, others result in inadvertent problems characteristic of an allergic reaction.

Eosinophilia

In the normal animal or human, eosinophils make up only a small percentage of the circulating white blood cells, usually <1,000/μL. Because eosinophil counts are often increased in metazoan parasitic or allergic states, it is likely that they play a role in combating these problems. Eosinophilia is present in acute and chronic diseases involving mast cell degranulation, parasitism with tissue migration or invasion, allergy, or inflammation in tissues such as lungs and intestines which normally contain eosinophils. Examples include allergic bronchitis, eosinophilic gastroenteritis, trichinosis, flea-bite dermatitis, and cutaneous eosinophilic granuloma complex of cats. The level of circulating eosinophilia does not always correlate with the degree of tissue infiltration with eosinophils. Trichinosis, because of the extensive migration of larvae through the tissues, has been especially well studied, and much of what is known about eosinophil function comes from experimental infection of rodents with trichinae. Alternatively, parasites such as adult tapeworms are not likely to cause eosinophilia because minimal to no tissue invasion occurs.

In allergies, leukotriene C and platelet-activating factor stimulate smooth-muscle contraction, increase vascular permeability, and increase the release of histamine from mast cells.

Hypoadrenocorticism, known also as Addison's disease, has been found most commonly in humans and dogs. When the adrenal gland fails to produce enough mineralocorticoid and glucocorticoid, animals are unable to respond to the stresses of daily life and may quickly become very weak and experience other specific signs of illness. Usually when an animal is very ill for any reason, a glucocorticoid-mediated eosinopenia occurs, but animals with hypoadrenocorticism are unable to do this. So a very sick animal with normal to increased lymphocyte and eosinophil counts should be evaluated for this disease.

A group of lung disorders in a variety of species has been called *pulmonary infiltrates with eosinophilia,* or *PIE syndrome.* The cause is unknown, although a reaction to some undefined allergen might be present in some affected individuals. The term *hypereosinophilic syndrome* is used to describe a systemic disease most commonly seen in cats and associated with moderate to severe circulating eosinophilia and infiltration of multiple tissues, especially the gastrointestinal tract and lungs, with eosinophils. The intestines may become so thickened from the eosinophilic infiltrate that malabsorption results. At times it is difficult to say whether the condition is reactive to some specific stimulus or whether it may be a malignant proliferation of eosinophils. Eosinophilia rarely is present in malignancies and granulomatous inflammatory diseases. Because eosinophilia or tissue infiltration with eosinophils sometimes occurs without an obvious explanation, some have described eosinophils as being associated with the 3 "W's": worms, wheezes (allergies), and weird diseases.

Eosinopenia

The most common cause of a decreased eosinophil count is administration of corticosteroids, which causes eosinopenia beginning 2–3 hours after administration. The duration varies with the type of steroid given. The reason for the drop in eosinophil numbers is initially a redistribution of eosinophils into capillary beds, and later reduced production. Eosinopenia is also a feature of hyperadrenocorticism because of increased endogenous corticosteroid concentration.

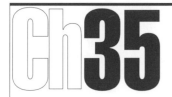

Basophils and Mast Cells

Canine Basophil

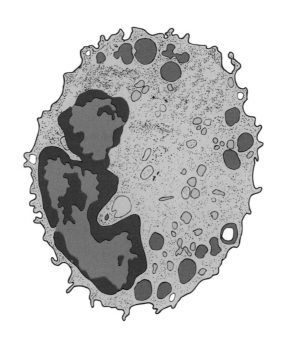

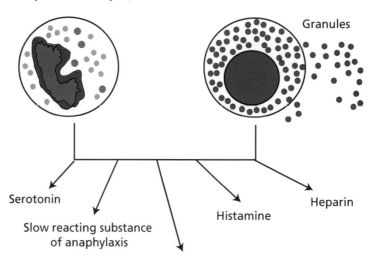

Basophil
(Fewer granules, nucleus like
eosinophil or neutrophil)

Mast cell
(Many granules, round nucleus)

Granules

Serotonin

Slow reacting substance
of anaphylaxis

Platelet–activating factor

Histamine

Heparin

Basophils frequently are equated with tissue mast cells because of some morphological and functional similarities, but the origin of each is not known for certain. It is not even known if they evolve from the same progenitor or if they each have their own progenitor. It is more likely that basophils are formed and mature in the marrow, and that mast cells are derived from pluripotent hematopoietic stem cells but undergo most of their differentiation in the tissues.

Basophils are rarely seen in the blood of healthy humans or animals, whereas mast cells are common in the tissues. The rabbit has relatively more circulating basophils (10%–15% of the total white cell number) and fewer tissue mast cells than most species. Ruminants are more likely to have circulating basophils than are dogs or cats. Mast cells are not normally present in the blood, although an occasional one may be seen on a concentrated (buffy coat) smear of centrifuged anticoagulated blood. Basophils are terminally differentiated and can no longer divide, whereas mast cells retain the ability to divide. Basophils circulate for a few hours and migrate to the tissues, where they may survive a few days. Mast cells can survive in the tissues from weeks to months. Mast cells are numerous in many tissues, but especially in the skin, subcutaneous tissues, lungs, pleura, peritoneum, mesentery, scrotum, uterus, and in the dog, the liver. Because the serosal linings of body cavities contain many mast cells, release of heparin may inhibit clotting of blood after hemorrhage into the cavity.

Appearance of Basophils and Mast Cells

The size of basophils is similar to that of eosinophils. As with eosinophils, the specific granules of basophils become visible at the myelocyte stage of development. The bluish color of the granules is caused by the high content of acid mucopolysaccharides, although the degree of color is variable between species. Cat basophils have violet granules in a gray cytoplasm, whereas basophils in most other domestic animals have granules of a darker color. The nucleus is multilobed and granules are relatively few. The contents of basophil granules are water soluble and may be dissolved during processing, making the cell difficult to identify. The mast cell has a round nucleus with small densely packed granules, even to the point of obscuring the nucleus (**Figure**).

Function

Basophils play a role in immune-mediated inflammation, especially anaphylaxis and cutaneous hypersensitivity, but specific stimuli are not well understood.

The granules of both basophils and mast cells are rich in histamine, heparin, serotonin, and hyaluronic acid. It has been estimated that the majority of the histamine in the body comes from these cells. After injury or antigen-antibody reactions, particularly those involving IgE in a sensitized animal, immediate degranulation of mast cells takes place. Histamine is released into the locality of the injury, resulting in smooth-muscle contraction, vasodilation, and leakage of fluid from the vessels. The effects of histamine vary with the specific type of histamine receptor in the tissue. For example, stimulation of H_1 receptors causes signs of acute allergic reaction or even anaphylaxis, whereas stimulation of H_2 receptors in the gastric mucosa causes increased secretion of hydrochloric acid, which over time causes gastric and duodenal ulceration. Activated mast cells and antibody-coated basophils elaborate IL-6, GM-CSF, and eosinophilic chemotaxic factor of anaphylaxis, which enhance inflammation, attract eosinophils and neutrophils to the site, and increase the production of additional white cells.

Both basophils and mast cells may be able to resynthesize granules, so they are not destroyed like neutrophils in the process of degranulation. Both cells are inhibited by corticosteroids, and the adverse effects of histamine may be suppressed by antihistamine H_1 blockers and specific blockers of the H_2 receptor.

Basophilia

Increases in basophil numbers are rarely numerically dramatic, but basophilia is associated with diseases causing increased IgE production, for example, heartworm in dogs. As a general rule, eosinophils and basophils respond to the same stimuli, and an increase in either probably has the same significance. Increases in eosinophils and basophils may be seen in dogs with disseminated mast cell tumor.

Basopenia

Because the basophil is rarely seen in the circulation, the absence of basophils is not recognized as abnormal.

Circulating Mast Cells

Mast cells normally are not present in the blood. Occasionally significant numbers are seen in the blood of dogs or cats with systemic mastocytosis (*see* Chapter 57). In these patients the marrow usually is partially replaced by malignant mast cells. Occasionally small numbers of mast cells enter the blood of animals with allergic diseases. Ordinarily, a buffy coat preparation of blood centrifuged in a capillary tube is needed to find small numbers.

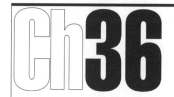

Lymphocytes

Production and Interaction of Lymphocytes

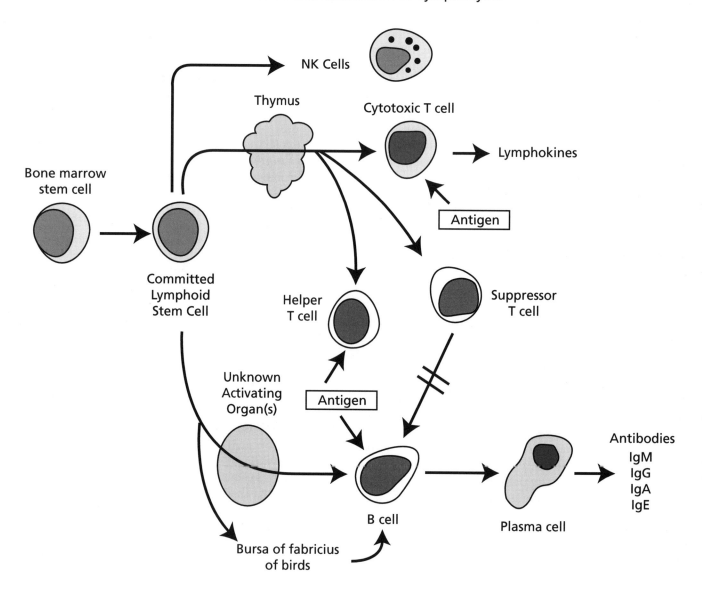

Lymphocytes are produced by pluripotent stem cells in the marrow; the production of lymphocytes branches off early from the rest of the hematopoietic progenitors. Some lymphocyte precursors migrate to the thymus where they acquire the ability to function as T cells. Others are processed further in the marrow and become B cells (**Figure**). Mature lymphocytes are found primarily in the lymphoid organs or in the lymphatic vessels (*see* Chapters 38–40). Lymphocytes continue to replicate after leaving the marrow. The life span of individual lymphocytes varies from a few days for some cytotoxic cells to many years for memory cells. After birth, most lymphocyte proliferation takes place outside of the marrow. Proliferation is driven by antigen and results in clonal expansion of lymphocytes that have surface receptors for the inciting antigen.

Structure

Most circulating lymphocytes are long-lived small lymphocytes 5–12 μ in diameter. The nucleus has coarsely clumped chromatin and is generally round but may be oval or slightly indented or cleaved. A nucleolus is not normally seen, and the amount of cytoplasm is scanty. The color of the cytoplasm is clear to light blue but may become darker blue in response to antigenic stimulation. Lymphocytes are capable of motility and chemotaxis, but to a much lesser extent than neutrophils.

The 2 functional classes of lymphocytes, B and T cells, are not distinguished morphologically by light microscopy, although they typically reside in different locations in lymphoid organs.

T Cells

Most circulating lymphocytes (about 65%–75%) are T cells. In addition, T cells predominate in paracortical regions of the thymus and lymph nodes. Lymphoid differentiation toward a T-cell lineage in the thymus is influenced by several thymic hormones. The stages of differentiation have been identified by the presence or absence of certain surface markers. Mature T cells display different cell-surface markers, depending on the specific subtype. Antibodies prepared to these markers are used not only to identify proportions of lymphocyte subsets, but also to classify malignancies of lymphoid origin. Some of these surface antigens, e.g., CD3 on T cells, involve antigen recognition. Helper T cells express CD4 whereas cytotoxic/suppressor T cells express CD8. Most circulating T cells in normal humans and animals are CD4 positive (CD4$^+$). The CD4 antigen also serves as a receptor for human or feline immunodeficiency viruses. Destruction of CD4-positive cells by virus causes immunosuppression. Helper T cells cooperate with B cells to stimulate their differentiation into plasma cells. IL-2 induces cytotoxic activity of other T cells as well as acts as a B-cell growth factor.

Cellular immunity is expressed primarily by T cells, which are responsible for delayed hypersensitivity, foreign graft rejection, graft-versus-host disease, cytotoxicity, and production of lymphokines. Cytotoxicity involves CD8$^+$ T cells in an antigen-dependent manner and

NK cells in an antigen-independent manner. Certain T cells also control or suppress antibody production.

Most lymphokines are produced by activated T cells. Commonly known lymphokines include various hematopoietic growth factors and interleukins that attract or activate other lymphocytes or white blood cells. IFNs are produced by T or B cells in response to bacterial, viral, or even chemical agents. If the thymus never develops or is destroyed, that animal lacks T cells and the ability to express cell-mediated immunity.

B Cells and Plasma Cells

In birds, a lymphoid organ, the bursa of Fabricius, participates in the processing of some undifferentiated lymphoid cells into B cells that have the ability to differentiate into plasma cells. In mammals, the marrow assumes the function of the bursa. B cells are found primarily in the germinal centers of the cortex of lymph nodes, the white pulp of the spleen, and the gut-associated lymphoid tissue. In response to a specific antigen, B cells proliferate, differentiate into plasma cells, and secrete an antibody specific for that antigen.

Plasma cells are oval with a round eccentric nucleus. The chromatin is clumped and arranged in a spoke-wheel pattern on fixed tissue specimens stained with hematoxylin and eosin. The cytoplasm stains deep blue with Wright's stain because of abundant ribosomes secreting immunoglobulin. A light perinuclear zone is a Golgi complex. Some plasma cells may have large red-purple inclusions in the cytoplasm (Russell bodies) containing antibody.

When antibody is produced to a new antigen, IgM is produced first, followed later by another class, usually IgG. In a primary encounter with an antigen, the switch from IgM to IgG, IgA, or IgE is governed at least partially by interactions with helper T cells. If this clone of B cells re-encounters the same antigen at a later time, the response is more rapid and a heightened production of non-IgM antibody occurs. This response is referred to as a *secondary* or *anamnestic response*. Plasma cells rarely are seen in the blood of healthy animals, but are common in the spleen and lymph nodes. An increased number of plasma cells may occur in the bone marrow of animals with immune-mediated hematological disorders, of dogs with ehrlichiosis, and of animals with myeloma, a malignancy of plasma cells.

B cells can be identified by the presence of immunoglobulin, and other cell-surface markers.

Other Cells of the Lymphoid System

A population of null cells contains no identifiable markers of either T- or B-cell origin. These may be immature cells or even stem cells that enter the circulation.

NK cells appear as lymphocytes with azurophilic granules. They have the ability to kill abnormal cells such as tumor cells or virus-infected cells without requiring prior recognition or antibody. The origin of NK cells is not clear, although they have some similarities to T cells.

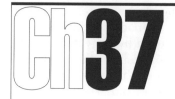

Patterns of Change in Lymphocyte Numbers

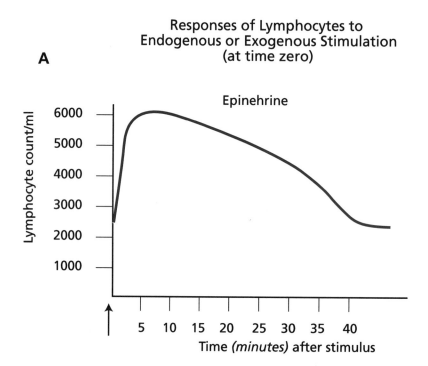

Responses of Lymphocytes to
Endogenous or Exogenous Stimulation
(at time zero)

A

Epinehrine

Lymphocyte count/ml

Time *(minutes)* after stimulus

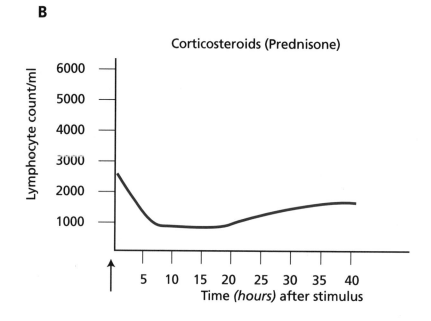

B

Corticosteroids (Prednisone)

Lymphocyte count/ml

Time *(hours)* after stimulus

74 Quick Look: Hematology

Lymphocytosis

The proportion of circulating white blood cells composed of lymphocytes varies with age and between species. Young animals normally have higher lymphocyte counts than do adults. Dogs and cats primarily have neutrophils in the circulation, whereas cattle, sheep, and goats primarily have lymphocytes, and horses have approximately half neutrophils and half lymphocytes. In the presence of inflammation, the ratio of lymphocytes to neutrophils may be reversed in ruminants.

Changes in lymphocyte number usually reflect changes in distribution or in recirculation rather than increased or decreased production. Lymphocytosis termed *physiological lymphocytosis* can occur secondary to epinephrine secretion (**Part A**). It usually occurs with neutrophilia when marginated cells are thrust into the circulating pool by increased systolic blood pressure during physical exercise or emotional excitement. The lymphocyte count can rise within seconds of a " fight-or-flight" reaction. It subsides within 30–60 minutes after the emergency is over. This response is often seen in young cats being restrained for blood to be drawn.

Reactive lymphocytosis may occur after antigenic stimulation, although this is not observed often in clinical practice. Reactive lymphocytes sometimes called *immunocytes* or *immunoblasts* are of B-cell origin. They can be recognized by their larger size and deep-blue cytoplasm. The color is produced by an increased density of ribosomes. Their presence in the circulation implies antigenic stimulation. Persistent lymphocytosis has been observed in cattle infected with bovine leukemia virus. The proliferation is a polyclonal proliferation of B cells and is reactive, not malignant. It does not appear to be a premalignant change. Reactive lymphocytosis does occur in the lymph nodes of animals responding to infection, immune-mediated diseases, or other antigenic stimulation. This nodal enlargement (lymphadenopathy) can be localized as in a patient with a dental abscess, or generalized, as in some systemic diseases.

Malignant proliferation of lymphocytes occurs in lymphoma or in leukemia of lymphoid origin. Chronic lymphocytic leukemia, discussed in Chapter 55, is associated with an increased number of normal- or near-normal-appearing lymphocytes. In the early stages of the disease it can be difficult to differentiate this from other causes of lymphocytosis. In acute lymphoblastic leukemia or lymphoma with marrow involvement, any malignant cells in the circulation would be morphologically immature and usually associated with other cytopenias.

Lymphopenia

Corticosteroids induce lymphopenia and eosinopenia in addition to neutrophilia and sometimes monocytosis (**Part B**). Part of the decrease in lymphocytes is due to redistribution from the blood to the tissues, and part to destruction of lymphocytes. The T cells seem to be especially sensitive to this steroid-induced lymphopenia. The effect begins within a few hours after an increase in endogenous steroid secretion or after exogenous administration, and lasts for hours to days depending on the steroid. Animals with severe injury or illness usually have a higher-than-normal concentration of endogenous steroids, resulting in a "glucocorticoid stress" leukogram: neutrophilia, lymphopenia, and eosinopenia. In fact, if an inflammatory disease is acute or overwhelming, neutropenia (sometimes with a left shift) may be present with lymphopenia and eosinopenia. The return of lymphocytes and eosinophils is regarded as a favorable prognostic sign.

Animals, particularly dogs, with adrenocortical hyperplasia (Cushing's disease) have persistent lymphopenia. Also, severely ill dogs with hypoadrenocorticism (Addison's disease) may first be suspected to have that diagnosis when a leukogram fails to show the expected lymphopenia and eosinopenia.

Lymphopenia from loss of lymphocytes and decreased production may occur after whole-body irradiation or anticancer chemotherapy. In these situations, neutropenia, perhaps with other cytopenias, may occur as well. Lymphopenia is often present in aplastic anemia. Foals with combined immunodeficiency disease are typically lymphopenic with aplasia of the thymus and lymph nodes.

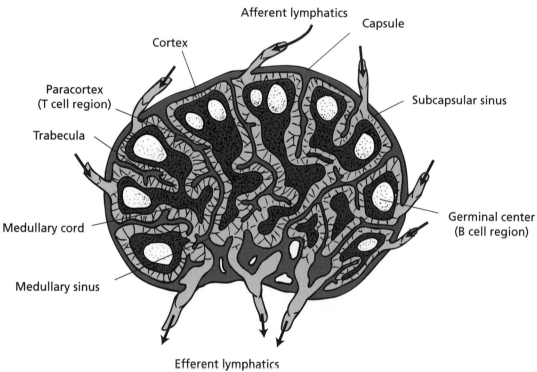

Normal Lymph Node

Afferent lymphatics
Capsule
Cortex
Paracortex (T cell region)
Trabecula
Subcapsular sinus
Medullary cord
Germinal center (B cell region)
Medullary sinus
Efferent lymphatics

Most T-cells reside in the paracortical regions.
Most B-cells reside in the germinal centers.

The lymphatic system arises from mesenchyme (mesoderm) as clefts that become lined by specialized mesenchymal cells (endothelium). Spaces dilate and coalesce to form central lymph sacs that unite and form 1-way (because of the internal valves) lymph channels. Lymph nodes become associated with these channels in mammals but not in birds or reptiles. The lymphatic system is independent of the blood vascular system except at the points where a major lymph vessel, the thoracic duct, empties into the subclavian vein near the heart. Lymphocytes can enter and leave the circulation many times during their life.

Lymphatic vessels are an adjunct to the venous system. They are not found in the brain, spinal cord, or skeletal muscle or within the bone marrow and splenic pulp. The primary functions of lymph nodes are phagocytosis, filtering foreign material and antigens from lymph drainage, and proliferation of B and T lymphocytes and plasma cells following exposure to immune stimuli associated with macrophage-lymphocyte contact with antigens.

Structure

The structure of a lymph node is shown in the **Figure**. The afferent lymph vessels enter the subcapsular sinus and proceed through the cortical and medullary sinuses to the efferent lymph vessels. Lymphocytes go from the blood to lymph nodes via the capsular and trabecular arteries, to the capillaries in the medullary cords, and then to postcapillary venules which have cuboidal endothelium that permits emigration of lymphocytes into the lymph node stroma. The cortex of porcine lymph nodes is centrally located, due to a peculiar anatomical folding of swine lymph nodes. Blood and lymphatic vessels similar to those in other mammals, penetrate into the cortex and the flow of fluids is identical to that of other mammals.

Any nonspecific enlargement of a single node or group of nodes is called *lymphadenopathy* or *lymphadenomegaly*. Nodes might be enlarged because of reactive hyperplasia secondary to an immune stimulation, causing proliferation of lymphocytes, or infiltration of neutrophils and macrophages caused by inflammation, or infiltration with neoplastic cells.

Reactive Hyperplasia

Young animals often show a variable degree of peripheral and visceral lymph node enlargement around the time of puberty. Tonsillar enlargement is also seen at this same time. This is considered normal and is not associated with clinical disease.

Infectious agents evoke the proliferation of T and B lymphocytes in addition to macrophages and monocytes. Minimal numbers of neutrophils are present with this type of response, which distinguishes reactive hyperplasia from inflammation that also might occur in response to bacterial infections. Increased numbers of lymphocytes and plasma cells are characteristic of hyperplasia.

A distinctive type of peripheral lymph node hyperplasia has been observed in cats between 6 months and 2 years old. A mixed population of lymphocytes and macrophages proliferates so much that the natural architecture of the node is no longer visible. Affected animals are often febrile with hepatosplenomegaly. About 50% are seropositive for feline leukemia virus. Some are infected with *Bartonella henselae,* the agent causing cat scratch disease in humans. Most animals recover, but a few develop lymphoma at a later time.

Lymphadenitis

An inflammatory response in a lymph node may be directed toward infectious agents or toxic insults. The pattern of inflammation is often quite specific, and such patterns are helpful in predicting the class of infectious agent involved.

Acute necrotizing inflammation can be caused by any acute, usually systemic bacterial infection, especially in young animals. Toxoplasmosis, a protozoal infection, also causes significant necrosis in affected nodes. Among bacterial infections, salmonellosis and tularemia typically cause necrosis.

Acute suppurative inflammation associated with a neutrophilic infiltration is caused by streptococci; *Corynebacterium* species, especially in sheep; *Pasteurella* bacteria, especially in rabbits; *Erysipelothrix* in swine; and *Rickettsiae*.

Histiocytic (macrophage) and plasmacytic lymphadenitis are likely to occur with infections such as histoplasmosis (fungus) and ehrlichiosis (rickettsia).

Granulomatous inflammation may be seen with infections such as tuberculosis, brucellosis, actinomycosis, leishmaniasis, feline infectious peritonitis, and some fungal infections.

Eosinophilic lymphadenitis might be seen with eosinophilic enteritis of horses, cats, and dogs; with feline hypereosinophilic syndrome; and secondary to allergies.

Neoplasia

Lymphomas (primary tumors of lymphoid tissue) are among the most common tumors in many animals such as dogs, cats, cattle, and poultry (*see* Chapter 53). Other tumors found in lymph nodes represent metastatic tumors from an area drained by the affected node(s). Malignant epithelial neoplasms more often metastasize to the regional nodes than do sarcomas, although both can metastasize by either lymphatics or veins. The regional nodes should be examined routinely during physical examination whenever there is a local inflammatory or neoplastic process. If malignancy is suspected, the regional node should be sampled or excised if it is enlarged. Most carcinomas begin growth in the subcapsular sinus. Nodal replacement by tumor may be so great that recognition of nodal tissue is difficult. Metastatic lesions in nodes may be larger than the primary tumor. The sublumbar nodes can be palpated rectally and should be examined whenever rectal, scrotal, or testicular neoplasia is suspected.

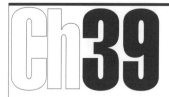

Thymus

Normal Thymus Gland: Young Animal

Low Power

A

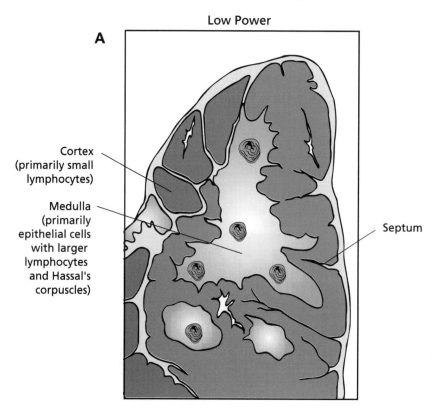

Cortex (primarily small lymphocytes)

Medulla (primarily epithelial cells with larger lymphocytes and Hassal's corpuscles)

Septum

High Power

B

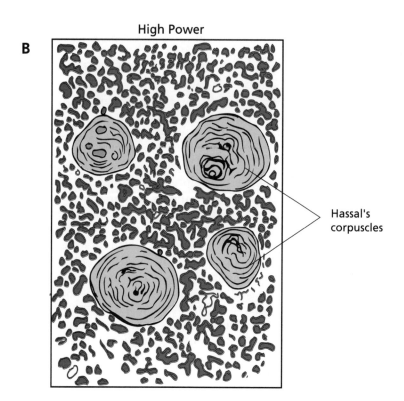

Hassal's corpuscles

The thymus is a bilobed ductless gland that arises from the endoderm of the ventral portion of the third and the fourth pharyngeal pouches. The 2 lobes become populated with lymphocytes of yolk sac and later bone marrow origin during the second month of gestation in humans. The thymic epithelium forms the framework of the glands and later the thymic corpuscles, which form during the third month of gestation. The 2 lobes join but do not fuse, and attach to and descend with the pericardial sac to lie within the thoracic cavity. Lobes and lobules within the gland are separated by fibrous Septae. The gland continues to enlarge until puberty and then atrophies. It never disappears, and traces of it can be found as thin wisps of tan tissue in the cranial mediastinum.

The cortex is composed primarily of small lymphocytes, and the medulla is composed of epithelial cells, which may be individual or in corpuscles (of Hassall) that keratinize, become cystic, or mineralize (**Parts A** and **B**). Lymphocytic follicles, sinuses, and afferent lymphatics are absent. Plasma cells are absent or rare in the thymus, but eosinophils and mast cells are seen sometimes and considered normal.

Anomalies

Congenital deviations from normal include aplasia, dysplasia, hypoplasia, and ectopia. Absence of a thymus (DiGeorge syndrome) is associated with immunodeficiency caused by an absence of T-cells. A strain of mice that lacks a thymus has been useful in the study of cell-mediated immune deficiency syndromes. These mice also lack hair (nude mouse). Since these mice readily accept grafts of foreign tissue, they are useful in cancer research. Tumors can be grown in these mice, and various treatments evaluated. A syndrome of combined immunodeficiency that includes thymic atrophy occurs in mice, Arabian horses, Basset hounds, and humans but is rare in other species.

Function

The primary function of the thymus concerns cell-mediated immunity, processing the various classes of T lymphocytes, the precursors of which migrate to the thymus from the marrow. The thymus also produces the hormones thymosin and thymopoietin.

Diseases

Cysts may be of thymic or pharyngeal pouch epithelial origin. Cysts are more common in cats and dogs with advancing age and are of no clinical significance.

Thymic atrophy occurs with some viral infections, particularly in kittens. These include feline leukemia virus, feline infectious peritonitis, and panleukopenia. Kittens can be born with a normal thymus that then regresses when these infections are acquired at a young age. Many animals die owing to profound immunosuppression. These disorders comprise part of the "fading kitten syndrome."

Primary tumors of the thymus arise from the epithelial component and are called *thymomas*. These tumors may be malignant or benign and occur in middle-aged and old animals as an anterior mediastinal mass. They must be distinguished from lymphomas, which also occur in this region. Thymomas tend to grow more slowly than lymphomas and are more likely to appear cystic on ultrasound examination. About 25% of canine thymomas are associated with signs of myasthenia gravis, a muscular disorder causing progressive weakness with exercise and paralysis of the esophagus. In humans, red cell aplasia has been associated with thymoma, but this has not yet been recognized in animals. Thymomas of cats are often well circumscribed and may be removed surgically, whereas those of dogs tend to be more invasive, and surgery is less often successful.

Spleen

Normal Spleen

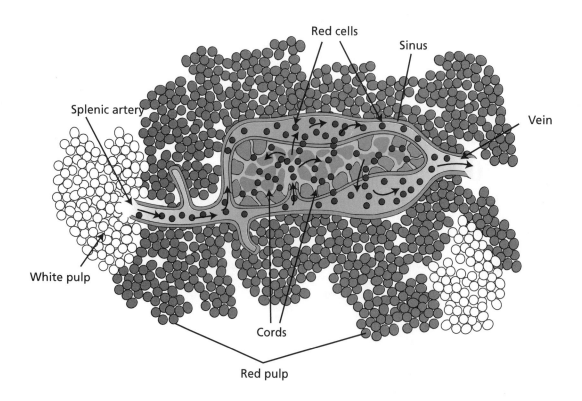

The splenic artery shown by the arrow passes through a sheath of lymphoid cells (white pulp), then penetrates into a loosely organized mass of phagocytes and reticular cells known as the splenic cords. Some branches of the splenic artery widen into sinuses (red pulp) and eventually join to form the splenic veins. Others end as open pipes that empty directly into the splenic cords.

The spleen arises from the mesoderm of the greater omentum as a series of masses beneath the surface epithelium. The masses fuse and slowly grow away from the greater omentum, which also forms the gastrosplenic ligament.

Functions

The marginal zones serve as filters of blood to remove old red cells or those coated with antibody. Sometimes only part of the antibody-coated red cell membrane is removed, leaving a spherocyte. Parasites or inclusions such as Heinz bodies or Howell-Jolly bodies are removed from red cells. Patients that have undergone splenectomy are at increased risk of infection with red cell parasites and some bacteria.

The spleen produces some lymphocytes and antibodies. Significant numbers of red cells and platelets are stored in the spleen and released when the spleen contracts in the presence of epinephrine. An animal that dies from hemorrhage will have a small spleen because the spleen is maximally contracted.

Anatomy

The circulation begins with the splenic artery to the trabecular artery through the white pulp to the sinus known as the *red pulp,* then to venous sinuses, trabecular veins, and finally the splenic vein. The splenic architecture is composed of the fibromuscular capsule and trabeculae; the red pulp, composed mainly of red cells; the cords of Billroth containing most of the macrophages, and sinuses; and the white pulp, composed primarily of lymphocytes (**Figure**).

The color varies with species and conditions. It might be cinnamon colored in the presence of splenic mast cell tumor. The spleen can take on the appearance of blackberry jam (black and soft) in animals with anthrax. Sometimes brown to gray capsular nodules called *siderofibrotic plaques* or red nodules composed of lymphocytic hyperplasia are observed as incidental findings at canine necropsy.

Diseases

The spleen is occasionally subject to traumatic rupture, and subsequent intra-abdominal hemorrhage can be fatal. Congested spleens or spleens with nodular lymphocytic hyperplasia are more friable and therefore subject to rupture from minimal trauma. *Splenosis* is a consequence of splenic rupture resulting in variably sized fragments of splenic tissue in the greater omentum.

Torsion of the spleen occasionally occurs in the canine and porcine species. The spleen becomes greatly enlarged owing to venous obstruction with variable patency in the arterial supply. Splenic torsion is a frequent complication of acute gastric dilatation with or without volvulus in the canine species. Animals with splenic torsion experience acute microangiopathic hemolysis.

The spleen can become diffusely enlarged (splenomegaly) from several causes. Passive congestion can occur as part of generalized circulatory failure or compromise of the portal circulation. Drugs such as barbiturates that may be used for euthanasia disrupt the smooth-muscle tone, causing splenomegaly, which is a common finding at necropsy.

Many chronic bacterial and viral infections cause splenomegaly. The reason for the enlargement is often reated to hyperplasia of lymphocytes and macrophages. Equine infectious anemia and some protozoal (babesiosis, malaria), rickettsial (anaplasmosis) and mycoplasma (haemobartonellosis) diseases cause splenomegaly. In addition to reactive hyperplasia, anemia can cause splenic enlargement from extramedullary hematopoiesis. Despite a valiant attempt, the spleen rarely produces enough functional hematopoietic cells to be of any benefit to the host. A cat with severe, prolonged anemia is especially prone to splenomegaly.

Thrombosis and infarction occur far more commonly than one would expect based on the microcirculation of the spleen. Splenic infarcts may vary from dark red when fresh, to dull, yellow or tan when a few days old. They commonly occur at the margins of the spleen. Disseminated intravascular coagulation can cause splenic infarcts as exemplified by swine with hog cholera and dogs with septicemia.

Malignancy

The dog and cat are the most often affected species. In most cases of splenomegaly secondary to a primary hematopoietic malignancy, the spleen is uniformly enlarged (*see* Chapters 53–55).

The most common primary splenic neoplasm is the hemangiosarcoma that occurs as a large mass on the spleen of large breeds of dogs such as German shepherds and golden retrievers. The right atrial appendage and retroperitoneal regions are other common sites for this very aggressive malignancy. Frequent sites of metastasis for this tumor include the lungs, liver, and brain. Most dogs initially present to their veterinarians because of sudden or episodic weakness associated with hemorrhage into the abdominal or pericardial cavities. Thrombosis with infarction and large areas of sinusoidal engorgement always occur with splenic hemangiosarcomas, resulting in the bulk of the enlargement being made up of blood, organized fibrin, and necrotic tissue.

Leiomyosarcoma, a primary tumor arising from smooth muscle, can occur in the spleen. Overall, approximately half of all large splenic masses in dogs are malignant; the rest are hematomas or infarcts. Splenectomy is the usual way to both diagnose and treat splenic masses, assuming that no evidence of metastatic disease is present.

Metastatic tumors occur occasionally in the spleen. The most common are mesenchymal in origin and include fibrosarcoma and osteosarcoma; the latter also can occur as a primary splenic tumor. Entrapment of epithelial malignancy in the spleen is rare.

Ch41 Endothelial Cells

Edothelial Function

A   To prevent coagulation

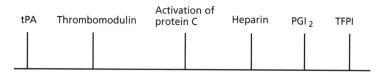

tPA | Thrombomodulin | Activation of protein C | Heparin | PGI₂ | TFPI

B   To stimulate coagulation

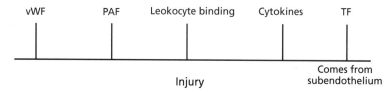

vWF | PAF | Leokocyte binding | Cytokines | TF

Injury

Comes from subendothelium

tPA = tissue plasminogen activator
PGI$_2$ = prostacyclin
TFPI = tissue factor pathway inhibitor
vWF = von Willebrand factor
PAF = platelet-activating factor
TF = Tissue factor

C   Interaction of Neutrophils with Endothelium in Inflammation

Random contact ⟶ Rolling ⟶ Sticking ⟶ Diapedesis ⟶ Chemotaxis

Selectins | Integrins

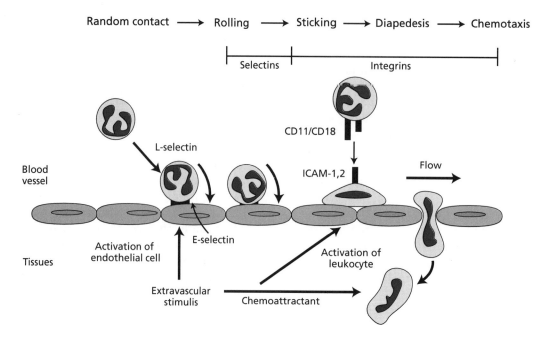

CD11/CD18

L-selectin

Blood vessel

ICAM-1,2

Flow

Activation of endothelial cell

E-selectin

Activation of leukocyte

Tissues

Extravascular stimulis

Chemoattractant

It has long been known that endothelial cells keep blood cells, some large molecules, and water in the vasculature. This view is overly simplistic as endothelial cells are among the most active in the body.

During embryonic development, endothelial cells come from a precursor called an *angioblast,* which is related to hematopoietic progenitors. In the adult, some endothelial cells have developed specialized properties. For example, renal endothelial cells are fenestrated to allow passage of certain substances between the blood and filtrate. In contrast, endothelial cells of the brain have tighter junctions that form the blood-brain barrier.

The endothelium regulates vascular smooth-muscle tone via vasodilators such as prostacyclin (PGI_2) and endothelium-derived relaxing factor (nitric oxide), and vasoconstrictors such as angiotensin II and endothelins. Endothelial cells also inactivate some vasoactive substances such as serotonin and bradykinin.

Prevention of Coagulation

In a normal animal, the endothelium makes and secretes substances that prevent blood from clotting (**Part A**). Endothelium provides a smooth barrier that prevents tissue factor (TF) in the subendothelium from coming in contact with clotting factors circulating in an inactive form. Antithrombotic factors of endothelial cells include prostacyclin (PGI_2), tissue factor pathway inhibitor (TFPI), tissue plasminogen activator (tPA), thrombomodulin, and heparin sulfate. PGI_2 produced by the cyclooxygenase pathway inhibits platelet aggregation. TFPI inhibits the activation of factors IX and X by the TF–factor VII complex. tPA is necessary for production of plasmin that breaks down fibrin. Heparin combines with antithrombin to inhibit thrombin. The interaction of thromboodulin with thrombin not only inactivates thrombin, but also activates protein C, which combines with protein S to inhibit fibrin production.

Coagulation

Stimulated by endothelial injury or inflammatory mediators, the endothelium changes to a procoagulant status and induces thrombus formation (**Part B**). TF combines with factor VII to activate the intrinsic and extrinsic coagulation pathways. The production of TF, plasminogen activator inhibitor, and von Willebrand factor (vWF) increases. Platelets adhere to damaged endothelium and to vWF and produce thromboxane, which causes platelet aggregation and vasoconstriction. Platelet-activating factor is produced by endothelium to recruit and activate more platelets.

Excessive activation of coagulation may be seen with extensive endothelial damage as occurs with heatstroke, with vasculitis, or in endothelial tumors such as hemangiosarcoma. This activation might result in disseminated intravascular coagulation, lung injury (ARDS), brain edema, or multiple-organ failure.

Inflammation

Injury, stress, cytokine release, and exposure to bacterial products produce marked changes in the structure and function of the endothelium. Local vasodilation results in increased blood flow and delivery of leukocytes to the site. Macrophages release TNF and IL-1 which cause edema secondary to elevated levels of endothelial cytoplasmic free calcium. This causes retraction of endothelial cells and leakage of fluid into the interstitial spaces. Leakage facilitates the egress of antibacterial substances and neutrophils to the site of inflammation, but excessive leakage of fluid into vital tissues such as the brain or lungs can be devastating.

Margination of neutrophils increases in response to endotoxin. Adhesion molecules on both leukocytes and endothelial cells cause initial rolling of blood cells, then adhesion, and diapedesis (**Part C**).

The initial binding is mediated by receptors on the neutrophil membranes, L- (leukocyte) selectins, that bind to endothelial cells. At the same time P- (platelet) and E- (endothelial) selectins become expressed when the endothelium encounters IL-1 or TNF from mononuclear phagocytes. Tighter binding by integrin molecules (CD11 and CD18) on neutrophils to intercellular adhesion molecules (ICAM-1 and -2), vascular cell adhesion molecule-1 (VCAM-1), and platelet-activating factor, all expressed by endothelial cells, follows. The density of these adhesion molecules is determined by the intensity of the inflammatory stimulus and the concentration of histamine, activated complement, and thrombin in the initial stages of inflammation. As a by-product of these events, oxygen radicals, and other neutrophil by-products, can cause endothelial damage.

Endothelial cells also play a role in cell-mediated immune reactions. Under the influence of IFN-γ, endothelial cells express the class II histocompatibility antigens necessary for antigen presentation to T cells. Migration of T and B cells into the tissues is also dependent on binding to receptors on endothelial cells.

Angiogenesis

Like other tissues of the body, endothelial cells need to repair damage and to proliferate into other growing tissues. In normal tissue growth and healing, angiogenic factors are released from ischemic or rapidly growing tissues. Examples of these factors are vascular endothelial cell growth factor (VEGF), basic fibroblast growth factor, and platelet-derived growth factor (PDGF). Heparin potentiates the effects of fibroblast growth factor and is important in the healing of wounds. New vessels sprout from small venules or occasionally capillaries.

Angiogenesis is a major factor in the progression and metastasis of malignant cells. Blood vessels are necessary for the growth of tumors to >2 mm in diameter. The prognosis for some tumors can be predicted by the degree of vascularization seen histologically. The metastatic cascade involves initial tumor growth, angiogenesis, and release of matrix-degrading metalloproteinases, which facilitate invasion into surrounding tissues and vessels. The tumor cells must survive in the blood vessels, exit, and invade a new metastatic site. Some primary tumors such as osteosarcoma in dogs and humans secrete soluble inhibitors of angiogenesis that prevent vascularization of metastases. If the primary tumor is removed, the metastatic cells become vascularized and grow more rapidly.

Action of Platelets in Vessel Wall Injury

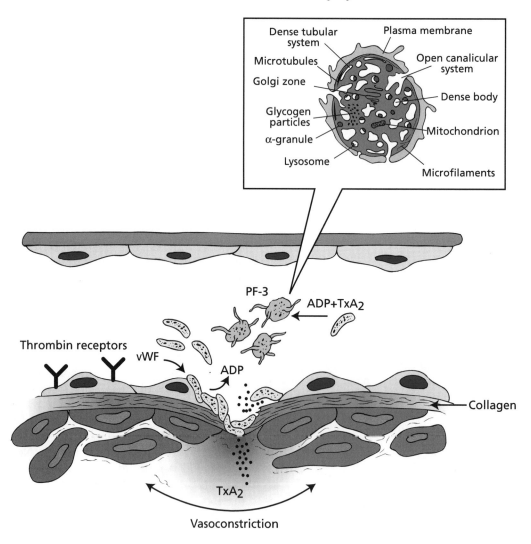

platelets are small fragments of the cytoplasm of megakaryocytes, which are large precursor cells in the marrow. They have no DNA and cannot synthesize new proteins. The role of platelets is to plug up small holes in vessels and help to initiate the formation of a fibrin clot.

Clotting of the blood requires precise interaction between platelets produced in the marrow and clotting factors, most of which are produced in the liver. The system of checks and balances necessary to keep the blood in a liquid state but prevent excessive bleeding is complex. The immediate response to endothelial damage is vasoconstriction, followed by formation of a platelet plug (primary hemostasis). This plug is then stabilized by formation of a fibrin clot (secondary hemostasis).

Platelets alone are adequate for plugging the "everyday," small pinpoint areas of damage that form in skin and mucous membranes. Fibrin is necessary to repair more severe damage.

Production

Megakaryocytes arise from the pluripotent stem cell. Under the stimulation of thrombopoietin, IL-3, IL-6, and GM-CSF, the multipotent progenitor becomes committed to the megakaryocyte line. The early megakaryocyte is larger than other blasts and has a round nucleus with a small amount of basophilic cytoplasm. The megakaryocyte grows by endomitosis, meaning that the DNA replicates without nuclear division. After 2–5 divisions the megakaryocyte is a very large cell with a multilobulated nucleus and small pink granules in the cytoplasm. Increased production of platelets can occur by increasing both the number of megakaryocytes and the number of platelets per megakaryocyte. As the megakaryocyte matures over several days, it differentiates, producing the granules and network of channels characteristic of platelets. Finally, individual platelets are demarcated and released by fragmentation while the nucleus is destroyed by macrophages. The platelets enter the circulation, where they remain for 7–10 days. When first released, young platelets are larger and function better than older platelets. Not all large platelets seen on a blood smear are young, however.

Circulation

As platelets circulate, they become smaller, and eventually they become less functional and are removed from the circulation. In the circulation the platelets do not interact with the endothelium unless damage occurs or they are activated by other mechanisms. At any one time, about two-thirds of the platelets are circulating and the rest are stored in the red pulp of the spleen. Splenic contraction during excitement or exercise releases additional platelets into the circulation.

Structure

Platelets are normally disk shaped, anucleated structures with a complex system of granules and tubules (**Figure**).

The plasma membrane contains adhesion molecules that bind to an injured endothelial surface. Receptors on the membrane also bind to thrombin, and to vWF. The membrane serves as a source of arachidonic acid that generates thromboxane A_2 (TxA_2) and other products of the cyclooxygenase pathway. Phospholipids in the membrane, referred to as *platelet factor 3* (PF-3), are necessary for the interaction with coagulation factors and calcium to form a fibrin clot.

The platelet matrix is located just beneath the platelet membrane and includes the contractile microfilaments actin and myosin and microtubules. The internal structure is composed of both dense granules that contain ADP (a potent platelet agonist), Ca^{2+}, ATP, and serotonin, and α-granules that contain glycoproteins, vWF, fibrinogen, and fibronectin.

Within the platelet is an open canalicular system that transports agonists inward and moves products of the platelet storage granules to the outside. In addition, a dense tubular system contains calcium and enzymes involved with prostaglandin synthesis.

Function

Platelet function is integral to the initiation and maintenance of hemostasis. The sequence of events is adhesion of platelets to damaged endothelium, aggregation with other platelets, and activation with release of the contents of granules. (see **Figure**). Platelet adhesion is mediated by vWF. If vWF is absent or nonfunctional, adhesion cannot occur even though the platelet itself is normal. The platelets change shape from a discoid or spherical to form pseudopods, and the granules become concentrated in the central portion of the platelet.

Following adhesion, platelet aggregation is stimulated by direct activation of platelets by exposure to collagen, thrombin, TxA_2, and epinephrine, which in combination with ADP recruit more platelets. Platelet aggregates are formed chiefly through platelet-platelet bridging. The ADP initially comes from the endothelium and then from the platelets themselves.

Platelet activation occurs as the platelets adhering to an injured endothelial surface release contents of α-granules and dense granules. Concurrently, platelets interact with the coagulation proteins, leading to the formation of thrombin and generation of a fibrin clot.

The platelet phospholipid surface is involved at several steps in the coagulation cascade. Platelet phospholipid maximizes the conversion of prothrombin to thrombin by providing a surface on which the complex of calcium and activated factors X and V can be formed efficiently.

Platelet aggregates eventually undergo a retraction process through a continuous cycle of pseudopod extension along fibrin strands and through actin-myosin contractions. Several hours after a clot forms, it contracts; this can be observed in vitro.

Coagulation

A

Fibrin Formation

Red blood cells

TF:VII

Ca^{++}

X

Fibrinogen

Xa

Fibrin

XIIa+XIa → IXa

VIIIa

PT → Fibrin

Fibrin

Va

Th

Endothelial cell

Fibrin strands

Platelets

Hemostatic events associated with vessel wall injury. These involve the organization of platelet plugs and fibrin deposition.

B

The Coagulaton Pathway

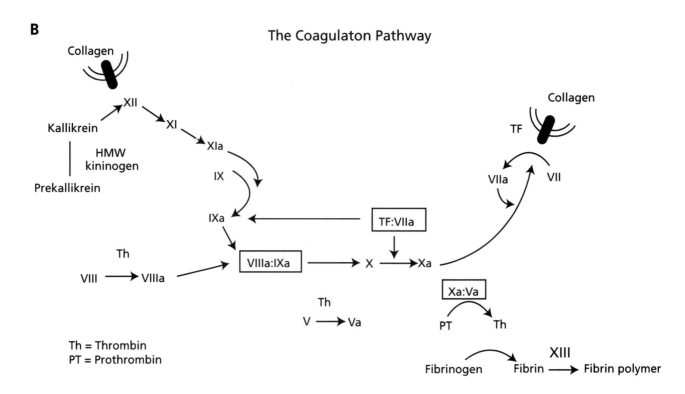

Collagen

XII

Kallikrein

XI

HMW kininogen

XIa

Prekallikrein

IX

IXa

Th

VIII → VIIIa

VIIIa:IXa

Collagen

TF

VIIa   VII

TF:VIIa

X → Xa

Th

V → Va

Xa:Va

PT → Th

Th = Thrombin
PT = Prothrombin

XIII

Fibrinogen → Fibrin → Fibrin polymer

Hemostasis is achieved through finely balanced interactions between blood flow, the vascular endothelium, platelets, and the production and clearance of coagulation and fibrinolytic factors, cofactors, and their inhibitors. Intact endothelial surfaces inhibit clotting, but damaged endothelial cells promote coagulation by activating platelets and by allowing exposure of circulating coagulation factors to TF. By exposing TF to circulating factor VII, endothelial injury triggers a sequence of reactions leading to the formation of a fibrin network that stabilizes and anchors the platelet plug. Concurrent with activation of the coagulation reactions, several natural anticoagulant systems aid in limiting clot formation to the site of injury. Other proteins function to slowly degrade the fibrin clot as healing ensues.

Fibrin Formation

TF is produced by subendothelial collagen and by activated monocytes, endothelial cells, and platelets. Exposure of TF to circulating factor VII initiates the process of fibrin formation. Fibrin is not present as such in the circulation but is produced from a precursor, fibrinogen. All of the other factors are proteins circulating as inactive precursors in the plasma. Fibrin formation involves a series of reactions. The products of each reaction catalyze a subsequent reaction or feed back to catalyze a previous reaction. The current scheme of coagulation places the TF–factor VII complex (TF:VII) in the role of initiating fibrin formation. In every case, the inactive form is activated by the cleavage of 1 or 2 peptide bonds.

The common names are generally used for factors I through IV (fibrinogen, prothrombin, TF, and calcium, respectively), and the Roman numeral designations are used for factors V and VII through XIII (there is no factor VI). The lowercase letter "a" is used to denote the active form of the factors. For example, factor II is prothrombin and factor IIa is thrombin. Except for TF and calcium, the major site of synthesis for most coagulation factors is the liver. Factor VIII circulates bound to a molecule, vWF, necessary for normal platelet adhesion to injured endothelium. To distinguish between the components of this complex, factor VIII coagulation factor is sometimes referred to as VIII:C, whereas vWF may be referred to as VIII:vWF. Factor VIII:C is a sex-linked gene product that acts as a cofactor in the activation of factor X. This seemingly minor cofactor role is actually critical to normal coagulation since the absence of factor VIII:C causes one of the most severe coagulopathies, hemophilia A. Endothelial cells and megakaryocytes produce the vWF portion of the factor VIII complex.

Although the biological half-life of each coagulation factor has not been established for each species of animal, it is slightly shorter than that reported in humans. In general the reported half-life of each factor can be placed into 1 of the following groups: 4–6 hours, factor VII; 12–24 hours, factors V, VIII, IX, and X; and 48–72 hours, fibrinogen, prothrombin, and factors XI and XII.

Coagulation Pathways

Coagulation is initiated by the exposure of TF to circulating factor VII and the formation of a factor VIIa–TF complex (TF:VIIa) (**Part A**). Factor VIIa probably exists in low concentration in plasma. TF:VIIa activates factor X. The process beginning with TF:VIIa is known as the *extrinsic pathway* since it starts with TF, which is primarily outside of the vasculature. The rest of the pathway from factor Xa to fibrin is the *common pathway*.

At the same time that TF:VIIa activates factor X, it also activates factor IX. Factor IX also can be activated slowly by exposure of factors XII and XI to a collagen or other rough surface. Factor XII is activated by contact with collagen. Kallikrein and high-molecular-weight kininogen also participate in the activation of factor XII and subsequently factor XI. The activation of factor XI is sometimes called the *contact phase of coagulation*. Since factor IX can be activated directly by TF:VII, factors XII and XI play a minor role in coagulation. Factor IXa, in combination with Ca^{2+}, (PF-3) and factor VIII, forms the intrinsic pathway, which also activates factor X. Factor Xa increases the rate of activation of factor VII and further activates factor IX. The prothrombinase complex is composed of factor Xa, factor V, Ca^{2+}, and PF-3. The prothrombinase complex acts on prothrombin to form thrombin. Thrombin cleaves fibrinopeptides from fibrinogen, forming a fibrin monomer. Feedback of thrombin also activates additional coagulation factors to produce additional thrombin. Fibrin monomers associate in an end-to-end and side-to-side manner to create fibrin polymers. Factor XIII, activated by thrombin to XIIIa, covalently cross-links the fibrin polymers into a stable clot (**Part B**).

Vitamin K–dependent Coagulation Factors

Vitamin K is a fat-soluble vitamin that comes mostly from the diet, but some is produced by bacterial synthesis in the intestines. Vitamin K serves as an essential cofactor for the synthesis of functional prothrombin, and factors VII, IX, and X; as well as the anti-coagulant proteins C and S. Normal function of these factors is dependent on γ-carboxylation of their terminal glutamate residues. Carboxylation of the vitamin K–dependent factors results in an overall negative charge, which allows them to bind calcium and interact with cellular membranes. Thus, vitamin K is not involved in the synthesis of the factors but is necessary for postsynthetic transformation in the liver. If vitamin K is missing for any reason, the liver still produces the vitamin K–dependent coagulation proteins, but they are not functional.

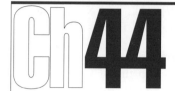
Anticoagulant Effects

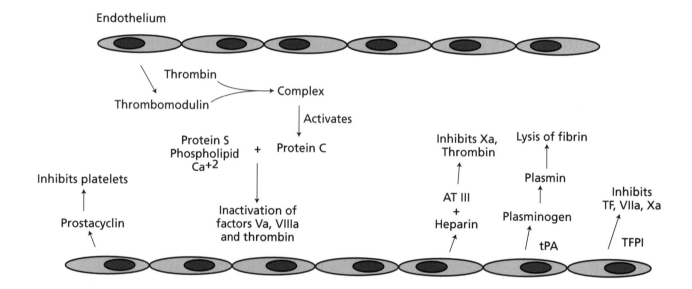

Endothelium

Thrombin

Thrombomodulin → Complex

Activates

Protein S
Phospholipid
Ca+2   +   Protein C

Inhibits Xa,
Thrombin

Lysis of fibrin

Inhibits platelets

Plasmin

Prostacyclin

AT III
+
Heparin

Plasminogen

Inhibits
TF, VIIa, Xa

Inactivation of
factors Va, VIIIa
and thrombin

tPA

TFPI

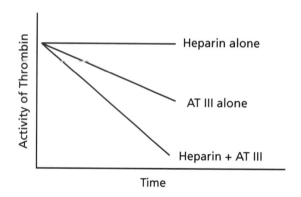

Activity of Thrombin

Heparin alone

AT III alone

Heparin + AT III

Time

Prevention of coagulation is just as important as coagulation. Blood must not coagulate as it circulates through the body. Natural anticoagulant systems also limit local coagulation after injury by inactivating coagulation factors and dissolving clots. The several inhibitor systems are either produced by endothelial cells or activated on endothelium. Some act primarily to eliminate activated coagulation factors and some act to destroy the fibrin clot (fibrinolysis) (**Figure**). Activated clotting factors can be removed by the liver or they can be inactivated directly in the plasma by the 3 natural anticoagulant systems described below. Additional inhibitors such as PGI_2 interfere with platelet function, and α_2-macroglobulin has a weak antithrombin effect.

TFPI

TFPI is an inhibitor that targets TF:VII complex and factor Xa, thus appearing to provide the regulating mechanism for the initiation of coagulation. TFPI circulates bound to plasma lipoproteins. The cell responsible for the production of TFPI is not known.

The Heparin–Antithrombin III System

Heparin-like molecules have been demonstrated on the luminal surface of the endothelium. These molecules act as a cofactor which binds to antithrombin III to greatly accelerate the formation of thrombin–antithrombin III complexes (see **Figure**). Antithrombin III (AT III), a glycoprotein, is a serine protease inhibitor produced by endothelium, megakaryocytes, and the liver. Antithrombins I and II do not exist. AT III functions to irreversibly inactivate thrombin and several other factors. Most activated clotting factors are serine proteases. After formation of the AT III–clotting factor complex, the complex dissociates from the heparin-like molecules, which are recycled. Heparin is necessary for the binding of AT III to endothelial cells, but heparin by itself has no anticoagulant effect. Under steady-state conditions, the heparin–AT III complex provides a mechanism to downregulate coagulant reactions on the endothelium by inactivating thrombin and other clotting factors that would otherwise participate in fibrin formation.

Protein C–Protein S– Thrombomodulin System

Endothelial cells express a cell-surface protein, thrombomodulin, that acts as a cofactor for thrombin-mediated protein C activation. Activated protein C is a vitamin K–dependent plasma protein that has anticoagulant activity because of a high affinity for thrombin. Protein C activation involves formation of a reversible complex between thrombin and thrombomodulin that eliminates the coagulant activity of thrombin and further activates protein C. In the presence of calcium and platelet phospholipid, activated protein C combines with protein S to inactivate other clotting factors (specifically factors V and III). Protein C is complementary to AT III, each having the most efficacy against factors not inhibited by the other.

Fibrinolysis and Tissue Plasminogen Activator– Plasminogen System

Physiological fibrinolysis is a process in which the insoluble fibrin clot is enzymatically digested when its usefulness is over. Fibrinolysis occurs at a slow rate that is synchronized with the healing of traumatized tissue. The mediator of fibrinolysis is the serine protease plasmin, which is formed from the inactive precursor plasminogen. The rate of plasmin generation is controlled by a delicate balance between plasminogen activators and plasmin inhibitors. The production of free plasmin in circulation is normally inhibited by several inhibitors including α_2-macroglobulin, α_1-antiplasmin, and AT III. Plasminogen can be activated to plasmin by the release of tissue plasminogen activator (tPA) from endothelial cells, which activates primarily plasminogen bound to fibrin in a clot. Alternatively, urokinase produced by kidney cells and secreted in the urine will activate plasminogen in the absence of fibrin. The value to the animal is that the risk of clots in the ureters is minimized. A similar polypeptide, streptokinase, is produced by streptococcal bacteria. Streptokinase, urokinase, and tPA are used clinically to treat thrombotic disorders. In addition, fibrin in the clot adsorbs circulating plasminogen, which is then activated by one of many plasminogen activators in the circulation or secreted by endothelial cells. Plasmin cleaves fibrin, generating a number of fragments called *fibrin-degradation products* (FDPs) or *fibrin-split products* (FSPs). The digestion of fibrinogen results in the production of FDPs, which bind thrombin and inhibit formation of a stable fibrin clot, thereby acting as potent anticoagulants. The FDPs also inhibit fibrin polymerization and interfere with platelet function. Normally the quantity of FDPs in the circulation is too small to play a major anticoagulant role, but in certain diseases the number can increase enough to increase the risk of bleeding.

Plasmin also plays a role in inflammation through interaction with complement, activated factor XII, kallikrein, and kinins.

PGI_2

Endothelial cells release arachidonic acid from the cell membrane through the action of phospholipases. In endothelial cells, PGI_2 synthetase converts arachidonic acid to PGI_2, the most powerful known inhibitor of platelet activation.

α_2-Macroglobulin

The only other plasma inhibitor of significance is α_2-macroglobulin, which is a weak protease inhibitor. It has some antithrombin and antiplasmin activities.

Testing of Coagulation

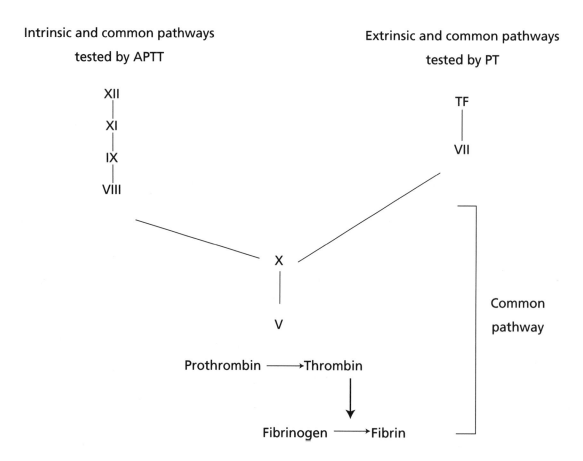

Intrinsic and common pathways
tested by APTT

XII
|
XI
|
IX
|
VIII

Extrinsic and common pathways
tested by PT

TF
|
VII

X

V

Common
pathway

Prothrombin ⟶ Thrombin

Fibrinogen ⟶ Fibrin

For the activated partial thrombosis time (APTT) to be normal, the intrinsic and common pathways must be normal. For the prothrombin time (PT) to be normal, the extrinsic and common pathways must be normal

Evaluation of the number of platelets, as well as the function of platelets and clotting factors, is necessary when a coagulation problem is suspected. Quantitative evaluation of individual clotting factors is done only in specialized labs. For coagulation to proceed normally, the body needs only a fraction of the platelets and concentration of clotting factors present in a normal animal. For example, the bleeding time, which tests platelet function, does not change until the platelet count drops to <100,000/µL, fewer than half of the normal number. Prothrombin time (PT) and activated partial thromboplastin time (APTT), tests of coagulation factors, become prolonged only when the concentration drops to <30% of normal. In one sense, the tests are not sensitive to early abnormalities, but an abnormality does tend to correlate well with clinical risk of bleeding.

Faulty venipuncture technique is a common cause of abnormal coagulation test results. Plasma containing TF and hemolyzed red cells rapidly activate clotting. The blood specimen to be tested should be obtained with minimal probing for the vessel. The blood sample should be centrifuged, and the plasma removed quickly for testing. Blood cannot be collected from catheters through which heparin has been administered or flushed. The preferred anticoagulant is 3.8% sodium citrate, which binds calcium. EDTA cannot be used as an anticoagulant for coagulation testing because it will chelate calcium irreversibly. Reference ranges for clotting tests are listed for common domestic species (see Chapter 58).

Platelet Tests

Platelet Count

Determination of platelet number is an important part of the initial evaluation of any animal with signs of abnormal bleeding. Estimation of a platelet count may be done during evaluation of the blood smear. Each platelet in a field examined using the 100 × oil immersion objective is equivalent to 15,000 platelets/µl of blood. For example, if an average of 20 platelets is seen per field, 20 × 15,000 equals an estimated count of 300,000/µl. Manual platelet counts are routinely performed on cats since they have large platelets normally and these may be mistaken for other cells on semiautomated counts. For most domestic species, platelet counts <100,000/µL are significantly low.

Bleeding Time

The buccal mucosa bleeding time has been determined for dogs and cats and appears to be a fairly reliable indicator of platelet function. In this test, a small puncture is made in buccal mucosa, and the time until clotting is noted. Thrombocytopenia will prolong the bleeding time so the platelet count should be >100,000/µL before this test is performed.

Coagulation Tests

Activated Clotting Time (ACT)

The ACT is useful to screen for abnormalities in the intrinsic or common pathway. The test uses a special tube that contains siliceous earth to ensure maximal exposure of blood to negatively charged surfaces and maximal activation of the intrinsic cascade. Whole blood is placed in the tube, mixed, and placed in a 37°C bath. The tube is removed at 30-second intervals, tilted, and examined for evidence of clot formation. A prolonged ACT indicates deficiencies in the intrinsic or common pathway. Since platelets provide the phospholipid necessary to support coagulation, severe thrombocytopenia (<10,000/µL) may prolong the ACT.

PT

This test measures the functional status of the extrinsic (factor VII:TF) and common (factors X and V, prothrombin, fibrinogen) pathways (**Figure**). Citrated plasma is added to a thromboplastin-calcium mixture, and the length of time required to form a fibrin clot is determined. Phospholipid is present in the reagent, making the test independent of platelet function. Due to the short half-life of factor VII, the test is very sensitive to vitamin K deficiency.

APTT (or PTT)

This test measures the functional status of factors in the intrinsic (XII, XI, IX, VIII) and common pathways. Citrated plasma is incubated with an activator of factor XII (kaolin) and cephaloplastins, which substitute for platelet phospholipid. Calcium is added, and the time required to form a fibrin clot is determined. Deficiencies of factor XII and kallikrein will prolong the APTT without associated hemorrhage.

Fibrinogen Concentration (mg/dL) Measured by Thrombin Time

When thrombin is added to plasma, fibrinogen is converted enzymatically to fibrin, which undergoes polymerization to form a fibrin network. The concentration of fibrinogen is determined from a standard curve. Fibrinogen levels may be decreased in some acquired or rarely congenital coagulopathies. They may be increased in inflammatory diseases.

Test for Fibrin and FDPs

The test (Thrombo-Wellcotest) involves a plate agglutination method using latex particles coated with antibody that causes agglutination in the presence of fibrin or fibrinogen fragments (FDPs). The presence of FDPs is abnormal and usually indicates ongoing fibrinolysis.

Specific testing is sometimes done to detect 1 of the fibrin fragments called *D-dimer*, which may be increased in thrombotic diseases.

von Willebrand Factor

Measurement of vWF should be considered for dogs with a suspected abnormality in platelet function and a normal platelet count. The test can also be run prior to breeding, to identify potential asymptomatic carriers of von Willebrand disease (vWD).

Evaluation of the Bleeding Patient

Interpretation of Test Results in
Disorders of Hemostasis

	Plt	PT	APTT	ACT	Fib	FDP	Confirming tests
Thrombocytopenia	↓	N	N	N or ↑	N	Negative	
DIC	↓	↑	↑	↑	↓	Positive	
Coumarin-type poison	N	↑	↑	↑	N	Negative[a]	Improved PT and APTT after treatment with vitamin K_1
vWD	N	N	N	N	N	Negative	↓ vWF ↑ Bleeding time
Factor VIII: C deficiency Factor IX deficiency Factor XI deficiency Factor XII deficiency– 　no clinical bleeding	N	N	↑	↑	N	Negative[a]	Specific factor assay–normal or ↑ vWF
Factor VII deficiency	N	↑	N	N	N	Negative	Specific factor assay
Factor X deficiency Prothrombin deficiency	N	↑	↑	↑	N	Negative	Specific factor assay
Platelet function defect	N	N	N	N	N	Negative	Platelet function tests ↑ Bleeding time
Myeloma with hyperglobulinemia	N or ↓[b]	N	N	N	N	Negative	Monoclonal gammopathy, Bone marrow: ↑ plasma cells

[a] FDPs may be detected if there has been major internal hemorrhage.
[b] May see low platelet count if marrow is extensively replaced by neoplastic cells.
Plt = Platelet count
Fib = Fibrinogen concentration
FDP = Fibrin/Fibrinogen = degradation products
N = Normal

The bleeding disorders of animals can be either inherited or acquired, the latter being more common. Inherited bleeding diseases are seen most often in rare breeds, which by necessity are inbred, and whenever particular animals are popular show-winners or sires and used extensively for breeding.

History

When confronted with a bleeding patient, one must first determine if a coagulopathy is present. Evidence of coagulopathy might include multiple petechiae or ecchymoses. A single large bruise might result from trauma and normal coagulation, or it might be associated with a coagulopathy. Epistaxis, melena, or hematuria is commonly observed in patients with a condition such as a nasal tumor, severe gastroenteritis, or cystitis, but also could be caused by thrombocytopenia. A clinician might suspect a coagulopathy if bleeding is more severe than expected, if it persists or recurs, or especially if bleeding is noted from >1 site.

Obtaining a complete medical history is an important part of the evaluation, and it should include information about the current and any previous episodes of bleeding, family history, environmental influences, and drug exposures.

Hereditary defects usually occur early in life, and affected animals may be stillborn or bleed at the time of birth. For others the first indication might be at the time of teething, during which any hemorrhage is abnormal. Surgical procedures such as neutering might be associated with hemorrhagic complications. Excessive bleeding after castration sometimes can lead to the diagnosis of X-linked diseases such as hemophilia A or B.

Acquired bleeding problems can occur at any age. If the patient was neutered without complications, a hereditary cause of bleeding is less likely. Young puppies are more likely to ingest toxins like warfarin, and the resulting hemorrhage might be confused with a hereditary coagulopathy.

A family history should be obtained whenever possible. Was a bleeding tendency present in relatives, and if so, was it spontaneous or secondary to trauma or surgery? Were both sexes affected, or were only males involved? Certain breeds are predisposed to specific inherited coagulopathies. For example, Doberman pinschers, Shetland Sheepdogs, and Scottish terriers, have an increased risk of vWD. Many breeds, and mixed breeds of dogs and occasionally cats, horses, and swine have developed hemophilia A. Even acquired coagulopathies may be seen more frequently in specific breeds, for example, immune-mediated thrombocytopenia (ITP) in cocker spaniels.

Environmental factors and exposures to drugs could be contributing factors. Pertinent information includes travel history to areas endemic for diseases such as ehrlichiosis, which causes thrombocytopenia. Also, does the animal roam freely, or is it confined? Is the owner aware of any rodenticides available in or near the home? Have any vaccines or drugs been administered recently? Modified live-virus vaccines may be a cause of ITP in dogs.

Tests may be indicated to rule out underlying diseases that could compromise hemostasis, e.g., uremia, autoimmune disease, malignancy, and systemic infections. Liver disease can result in decreased production of clotting factors.

Physical Examination

A thorough physical examination is essential to determine the location, severity, and nature of the bleeding and to identify any coexisting problems. The type and site of bleeding should be considered carefully. Platelet abnormalities are more likely to affect mucous membranes and skin. For example, epistaxis, hematuria, melena, petechiation, and ecchymosis, alone or in combination are usually associated with thrombocytopenia or abnormal platelet function. Clotting factor disorders are more likely to cause hematomas in soft tissues or bleeding into body cavities or joints.

Physical findings that suggest acquired rather than inherited causes are enlarged spleen, liver, or lymph nodes. Physical examination always should include a complete ocular examination to look for hyphema or retinal hemorrhages. Hyphema can occur with coagulopathies but also may be seen in dogs with lymphoma or uveitis with apparently normal coagulation.

A rectal examination might detect previously unnoticed gastrointestinal bleeding and perhaps give an indication of the site. Dark-red to black stools indicate bleeding proximal to the colon; the coloration could even be from swallowed blood from the nose or mouth in the presence or absence of a coagulation abnormality. Red blood generally comes from the colon or rectum. An ulcerated rectal mass might be palpable.

Lameness with single- or multiple-joint swelling could indicate inflammation, sepsis, or hemorrhage into joints.

Animals with thrombocytopenia secondary to bone marrow failure of any cause may have nonregenerative anemia or signs of sepsis because of neutropenia.

Laboratory Evaluation

A CBC including a platelet count provides information as to the presence of anemia and an evaluation of primary hemostasis (platelet number). In addition, the WBC count and morphology of all cell types might raise suspicion of bone marrow abnormality.

The rest of the coagulation profile includes the PT, APTT, fibrinogen concentration, and evaluation for FDPs (see Chapter 45). If these test results are not immediately available, an ACT can be used as a quick screen for intrinsic and common pathway abnormalities (Figure).

Additional tests, sometimes needed are a urinalysis, chemistry profile, and serological testing for retroviruses in cats or tick-borne diseases in dogs. If the clinical evaluation of the bleeding suggests a platelet abnormality and if the platelet count is not low enough to be the cause, a buccal mucosal bleeding time may be done to evaluate platelet function. Further testing of coagulation may require the help of specialized laboratories.

Causes of Thrombocytopenia and Thrombocytosis

Thrombocytopenia

A.. Inherited – e.g., cyclic hematopoiesis

B. Acquired

    1. Platelet destruction – most often immune mediated
        a. Primary – ITP
        b. Secondary – infections (e.g., ehrlichiosis),
           drugs, vaccines

    2. Platelet sequestration – e.g., conditions in which the
       spleen is enlarged

    3. Platelet consumption
        a. DIC from any cause – (e.g., hemangiosarcoma or
          other malignancies
        b. Vasculitis – e.g., Rocky Mountain spotted fever

    4. Decreased production
        a. Primary bone marrow diseases– e.g., aplastic anemia,
          hematopoietic malignancy
        b. Secondary to drugs – e.g., chloramphenicol,
          sulfonamides (antibacterial agents);
          phenylbutazone (anti-inflammatory agent);
          diphenylhydantoin (anticonvulsant); estrogen;
          chemotherapeutic drugs
        c. Secondary to infections – e.g., retroviruses

Thrombocytosis

A. Reactive – chronic bleeding

B. Essential thrombocythemia

Platelet disorders can be categorized quantitatively as *thrombocytopenia*, a platelet count less than the lower limit of the reference range, or *thrombocytosis*, a platelet count greater than the upper limit. Bleeding from platelet disorders is usually evident clinically as petechiae or ecchymoses in the skin or mucous membranes. Thrombocytopenia is much more common than defects in platelet function, and platelet counts usually are <20,000–30,000/μL before bleeding occurs, assuming platelet function and clotting factors are normal. Platelet counts of 30,000–100,000/μL may contribute to bleeding if a factor abnormality is also present. If the platelet count is >100,000/μL and if the platelets function normally (the bleeding time is normal), bleeding is not present.

Congenital thrombocytopenia is rare. Acquired thrombocytopenia can result from decreased platelet production or increased loss, sequestration, destruction, or consumption.

The typical clinical sign & thrombocytopenia is bleeding from small vessels in the skin or mucous membranes. These hemorrhages may be pinpoint (petechiae) or larger bruises (ecchymoses). Common sites of mucosal bleeding are the gingiva, nasal mucosa, and gastrointestinal or urinary tract. Anemia may result from blood loss. If surgery is performed, oozing from incision sites may be the first indication of a platelet-related coagulopathy.

ITP

The most common cause of severe thrombocytopenia in the dog is ITP. It has been found rarely in cats and horses and occurs in humans. Most affected dogs are middle-aged females or spayed females. Cocker spaniels are at increased risk, as are possibly poodles and old English sheepdogs. The signalment is similar to that in immune-mediated hemolytic anemia (IMHA). In fact, the 2 diseases may occur simultaneously (Evan's syndrome).

The classic presentation is that of petechiae or mucosal bleeding, in an otherwise healthy dog. The bleeding initially may be relatively mild despite *severe* thrombocytopenia. The platelet count is usually <10,000/μL and commonly <5000/μL. The antibody is directed against normal antigens (often IIb, IIIa) on the platelet membrane, resulting in removal of the platelets primarily by splenic macrophages. The same fate awaits any transfused normal platelets. Circulating platelets are often enlarged and function very well.

The number of megakaryocytes in the marrow in patients with ITP varies, depending on whether or not the antibody affects megakaryocytes. This is similar to the situation in IMHA, where the marrow may have erythroid hyperplasia or hypoplasia. Although the cause of ITP is usually unknown, the same syndrome may occur following vaccination with modified live-virus vaccines and perhaps from a viral infection.

Laboratory diagnosis of ITP is difficult, and the diagnosis is often made by excluding other causes of thrombocytopenia. Tests for antiplatelet antibodies are not used routinely.

Treatment of ITP, similar to that of IMHA, involves the use of corticosteroids alone or in combination with other immunosuppressive drugs. Most dogs recover with single or multiple courses of treatment.

Other Causes of Thrombocytopenia

Although ITP is the most common cause of severe thrombocytopenia, infectious diseases, drug or toxin exposures, consumption coagulopathy, and marrow diseases are also causative (**Figure**). Some infectious diseases such as ehrlichiosis in dogs, cause thrombocytopenia through destruction or consumption or decreased production of platelets. Ehrlichiosis occurs with a variable prevalence worldwide in dogs, and both monocytic and granulocytic ehrlichiosis can cause thrombocytopenia. Cats rarely are affected. In horses, *E. equi* causes thrombocytopenia, fever, anemia, and edema, whereas *Ehrlichia risticii* (Potomac horse fever) causes fever, neutropenia, and diarrhea.

Mild to moderate thrombocytopenia is a common early manifestation of sepsis. The cause is early DIC or consumption by interaction with damaged endothelium. For example, Rocky Mountain spotted fever, is often associated with vasculitis and consumption of platelets. Feline leukemia virus may cause thrombocytopenia by suppression of the marrow. Bovine virus diarrhea frequently causes thrombocytopenia in affected cattle.

Thrombocytopenia is a major component of DIC, described in more detail in Chapter 50. In DIC, platelet counts are moderately decreased, usually not to the degree seen with ITP, but the results of other coagulation tests are abnormal as well. In microangiopathic hemolysis, platelets are sequestered and consumed at the location of the abnormal vasculature (e.g., hemangiosarcoma of the dog).

Whenever the spleen is large for any reason, platelets and other blood cells can become sequestered. This has been referred to as *hypersplenism*.

Severe hemorrhage, whether acute or chronic, is unlikely to cause thrombocytopenia because of the extra platelets stored in the spleen or other sites. In fact, thrombocytosis is more likely to occur, especially with chronic hemorrhage, because of increased platelet production.

Some drugs and toxins cause thrombocytopenia by destruction of platelets, most commonly by an immune-mediated mechanism, or by suppression of the marrow.

Neoplasia can cause thrombocytopenia secondary to DIC. Hematopoietic neoplasia may fill the marrow with malignant cells (myelophthisis) and inhibit platelet production. If thrombocytopenia is caused by decreased production of platelets in the marrow, leukopenia or nonregenerative anemia or both may be present.

Thrombocytosis

Thrombocytosis is encountered infrequently. The most common cause is probably a reactive thrombocytosis in response to hemorrhage. Thrombocytosis occasionally is seen with myeloproliferative disorders, especially in cats. The condition called *essential thrombocythemia* is associated with platelet counts often >1,000,000/μL. See Chapter 55.

Qualitative (Functional) Platelet Disorders

A   Attachment of Platelets to an Injured Surface by von Willebrand Factor (vWF)

B   Functional Disorders of Platelets

Inherited

1. vWD – platelets normal; defect in adhesion
2. Canine thrombopathia (Bassett hounds)
3. Thrombasthenia (Otterhounds)
4. Bovine thrombopathia (Simmental cattle)
5. Chédiak-Higashi syndrome

Acquired

1. Drug induced
    a. Receptor blockade or alteration in membrane charge or permeability (some tranquilizers, local anesthetics, penicillins)
    b. Impairment of signal transduction
    c. Inhibition of cyclooxygenase (aspirin, NSAIDs)
2. Plasma cell malignancies
3. Uremia
4. Hypothermia

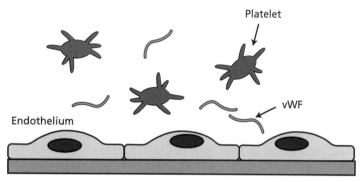

Platelet

vWF

Endothelium

Basement membrane

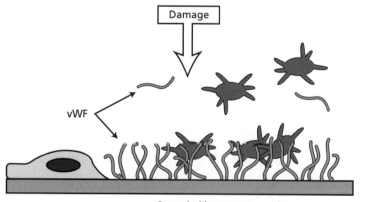

Damage

vWF

Denuded basement membrane

Qualitative disorders of platelets involve defects in adhesion, aggregation, or release of granule constitents, and are congenital or acquired.

ron Willebrand Disease (vWD)

vWD is the most common inherited coagulopathy in humans, pigs, and many breeds of dogs, especially the Doberman pinscher, Basset hound, standard poodle, Scottish terrier, golden retriever, German shepherd, and Shetland sheepdog. It is found rarely in cats and rabbits. vWD is inherited as an autosomal disorder characterized by abnormal or deficient vWF, normal or slightly prolonged APTT, and a normal platelet count. The condition is either dominant with incomplete penetrance, or recessive. vWF is a large multimeric glycoprotein synthesized in megakaryocytes and endothelial cells and found in plasma, platelets, and endothelial cells (**Part A**). It circulates as a complex with factor VIII, which it helps to stabilize. While the clinical presentation of vWD is one of compromised platelet function (i.e., mild to severe bleeding episodes generally involving mucosal surfaces rather than deep hemorrhage), the platelet itself is normal. The defect is one of diminished adhesion of platelets to damaged endothelium.

The severity of the clinical signs varies greatly. If the disease is mild, excessive bleeding might occur only after significant trauma or surgery, or after ingestion of drugs such as aspirin that adversely affect platelet function. Bleeding may occur following vaccination or during pregnancy or estrus. Cases may first be recognized because of excessive bleeding during teething, ear cropping, or neutering. Although severe vWD can cause death during the first few days of life, most cases are characterized by varying degrees of morbidity with minimal mortality.

Three types of the disease exist. Type 1 is the most common and is characterized by a variable decrease in all sizes of multimers of vWF. Type 1 vWD most commonly affects Doberman pinschers, although most are heterozygous and few have an increased tendency to bleed.

Type 2 disease is characterized by a depletion of high-molecular-weight multimers, which are most important for platelet adhesion. This type is more severe than type 1 and is seen in German shorthaired pointers.

Type 3 disease is characterized by the marked deficiency of all multimers and is inherited as a recessive trait. Clinically affected patients are homozygous, the offspring of 2 clinically normal heterozygotes. Type 3 vWD has been identified in Scottish terriers, Shetland sheepdogs, Chesapeake Bay retrievers, and Poland China swine and generally is the most severe form.

Diagnosis

The buccal mucosal bleeding time is often used as a screening test. Although it is not sensitive in detecting mild vWD, an increase in the bleeding time correlates fairly well with the tendency to bleed. The bleeding time also is not specific for vWD; any significant abnormality in platelet function will cause it to be prolonged.

The quantity of vWF can be measured through an antibody-based method to detect an antigen (vWF. Ag) on the vWF protein. If the antigen level is low, electrophoresis can be performed to determine which type of vWD is present. Heterozygous carriers of vWD have levels of vWF that are between 15% and 60% of the levels in normal dogs. Carriers with normal bleeding times should not be bred but can be neutered safely.

Treatment

If surgery is necessary in a dog with vWD and a prolonged bleeding time (>5 minutes) or if spontaneous bleeding is occurring, vWF can be supplied by transfusion of concentrated vWF in the form of cryoprecipitate. If cryoprecipitate is not available, fresh-frozen plasma or even whole blood will supply additional vWF. Desamino-8-D-arginine vasopressin (DDAVP) may cause release of additional vWF from the endothelium and decrease the bleeding time in some dogs with type 1 vWD.

Other Inherited Disorders of Platelet Function

An autosomal recessive thrombopathia occurs in some Basset hounds. In this disorder, platelets fail to aggregate normally for reasons that are not well understood. An autosomally inherited thrombopathy similar to Glanzmann's thrombasthenia in humans has occurred in otterhounds. The defect appears to be a deficiency in the platelet binding sites IIb and IIIa necessary for aggregation and clot retraction. Other inherited disorders that affect platelet function are listed in **Part B**. Testing for these disorders is available only at a specialized laboratory.

Acquired Disorders of Platelet Function

Mechanisms involved with drug-related functional disorders are inhibition of receptor binding of agonists, inhibition of transduction of messages received at the platelet surface, and inhibition of platelet responses associated with decreased generation of thromboxane. Aspirin is the most notorious because the irreversible inhibition of cyclooxygenase interferes with the ability of the platelet to produce thromboxane. Other nonsteroidal anti-inflammatory drugs (NSAIDs) have similar, but transient effects. The reason why most individuals do not bleed after receiving aspirin (although the bleeding time may be prolonged) is that new functional platelets are being produced constantly. The effects of aspirin can be devastating in a patient with another coexisting coagulation abnormality.

Platelet function may be abnormal in patients with plasma cell malignancies (*see* Chapter 56.)

Hypothermia from any cause causes abnormal platelet function, probably by slowing the metabolic functions of the platelet. Simply warming the patient can shorten the bleeding time. Uremia interferes with platelet function by poorly understood mechanisms.

X-Linked Inheritance

Mating of carrier female to normal male

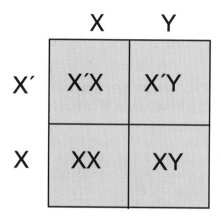

Offspring

Half of the females are normal

Half of the females are carriers

All females are assymptomatic

Half of the males are affected

Half of the males are normal

X′ – Chromosome carrying gene for hemophilia A or B

X – Normal X chromosome

Mating of carrier female to affected male

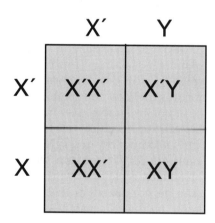

Offspring

Half of the females are affected

Half of the females are carriers

Half of the males are affected

Half of the males are normal

So long as one normal unaffected X chromosome is present the animal will not be clinically affected.

Bleeding in patients with clotting factor deficiencies occurs most commonly into areas of mechanical stress such as joints (hemarthroses), subcutaneous tissues, and muscles (hematomas). Bleeding also can occur into body cavities. Sometimes bleeding occurs into the brain or spinal cord, with devastating results. Bleeding can be delayed or recurring, as a platelet plug initially stops the bleeding but is washed away if a strong fibrin clot does not form.

Routine screening tests of clotting activity, such as the APTT, PT, and fibrinogen concentration, usually indicate whether a factor deficiency is in the intrinsic, extrinsic, or common pathway, but will not detect asymptomatic carriers. The reason is that heterozygotes have approximately half of the normal factor level, but the APTT and PT do not become abnormal until the concentration of a factor decreases to <30% of the normal amount.

Quantitative assays of specific clotting factors are necessary to identify the specific deficient factor in affected animals, and to screen normal relatives for the heterozygous state of such disorders. Carriers should be bred only if they are critical to a particular breeding program. Offspring of such planned matings can be tested for the defect in question. Those that are normal can be kept for breeding to maintain the blood line. Genetic counseling for animal breeders is an important responsibility of veterinarians.

Factor VII Deficiency

Factor VII deficiency has autosomal, incompletely dominant inheritance and has been found in several breeds of dogs. It is a mild disease with little or no clinical signs, other than easy bruising and an apparent predisposition to demodectic mange. The condition was discovered fortuitously by coagulation screening of beagles in commercial breeding stock before use in research studies. Homozygotes have prolonged PTs.

Factor VIII Deficiency (Hemophilia A)

Hemophilia A is a common and severe factor deficiency in humans and dogs, and recognized in horses, cats and cattle. An X chromosome–linked recessive disease, hemophilia A is carried by females and usually manifested in males (**Figure**). Female hemophiliacs can be produced by the mating of hemophiliac males to carrier females.

Mild cases frequently are undetected until the animal experiences teething, surgery, or trauma. Other cases are much more severe and detected at an early age, often when lameness occurs from bleeding into joints. Laboratory tests show a prolonged APTT. Affected animals have very low factor VIII coagulant activity (FVIII:C) but normal or elevated levels of vWF. Carrier, heterozygous females have concentrations of factor VIII that are about half of normal (40%–60%). Bleeding episodes can be controlled with cryoprecipitate prepared from fresh-frozen plasma. Because factor VIII has a relatively short half-life, treatment may have to be repeated.

Factor IX Deficiency (Hemophilia B)

Hemophilia B sometimes called *Christmas disease* tends to cause severe bleeding. An X chromosome–linked recessive disease like hemophilia A, hemophilia B has been found in dogs and cats, especially British shorthair cats. Results of diagnostic screening tests are the same as described for hemophilia A. A screening test to differentiate hemophilia A from B utilizes the fact that in the normal animal, factor VIII is consumed during coagulation whereas factor IX is not. Thus, normal serum contains factor IX but not VIII. An equal volume of normal serum is added to the plasma of a patient suspected to have hemophilia. The APTT will correct if factor IX is deficient, but not if factor VIII is deficient. For definitive results, however, concentrations of individual factors should be measured.

Factor X Deficiency

A rare autosomal disease recognized in American cocker spaniels, factor X deficiency results in severe bleeding in pups but is mild in adults unless they are subjected to surgery. The homozygous state of this condition is lethal. Surviving affected dogs are heterozygotes and have prolonged APTTs and PTs. Warfarin poisoning will cause similar test results and must be ruled out.

Factor XI Deficiency

Factor XI deficiency is an autosomal disease reported in dogs and cattle. Delayed bleeding occurs several hours after trauma or surgical procedures, but spontaneous bleeding is rare. Homozygotes have a prolonged APTTs.

Factor XII Deficiency

This autosomal condition has been recognized in some normal cats and dogs with a prolonged APTT. Thus this is a "laboratory disease," not a clinical problem for the patient. A low factor XII concentration is a normal physiological characteristic of marine mammals, reptiles, and birds.

Other Inherited Defects

Isolated families of boxers, otterhounds, and Devon Rex cats have had defects in the vitamin K–dependent synthesis or regulation of prothrombin-complex clotting factors. Laboratory findings, prolonged APTTs and PTs, are identical to those of warfarin poisoning, and administration of vitamin K corrects the problem (*see* Chapter 50).

An inherited prothrombin deficiency has been reported in English cocker spaniels. A family of Saanen dairy goats and several dogs with hereditary hypofibrinogenemia or abnormal function of fibrinogen have also been reported. Diagnostic tests in deficiencies of prothrombin or fibrinogen reveal a prolonged APTT and PT. To date no animals have been found to have either factor V or factor XIII deficiency.

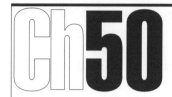

Pathogenesis of DIC

Tissue injury
Endothelial cell injury

Tissue factor expression

Platelet aggregation

Fibrin formation

Consumption of clotting factors, fibrinogen, and platelets

Activation of plasmin (fibrinolysis)

Microvascular occlusion

Bleeding

Fibrinogen and fibrin degradation products (FDP)

FDP's inhibit platelet aggregation fibrin polymerization thrombin

Vitamin K Deficiency and Antagonism

One of the most commonly encountered acquired coagulopathies in dogs and occasionally in cats results from interference with normal vitamin K metabolism by ingested rodenticides that contain warfarin or one of its derivatives. Dietary deficiency of vitamin K is virtually nonexistent in adult animals fed commercial diets. In newborn puppies, transient vitamin K deficiency occurs occasionally secondary to malnutrition of the bitch during gestation, and the immaturity of hepatic protein synthesis in the pup. Vitamin K and other fat-soluble vitamins are poorly absorbed in animals with chronic biliary obstruction or intestinal malabsorption syndromes, but only a small amount of vitamin K is necessary to sustain adequate synthesis of the vitamin K–dependent coagulation factors (II, VII, IX, X) and proteins C and S. Therefore, such syndromes must be well advanced and severe before a coagulopathy is manifested. Severe hepatic disease can result in a vitamin K deficiency. Drugs are infrequently incriminated in vitamin K antagonism; however, the use of antibiotics can destroy the normal gastrointestinal microflora that usually produce vitamin K. Cattle have been known to develop vitamin K antagonism by ingesting sweet clover hay, which contains a mold that produces a warfarin-like metabolite.

In warfarin toxicity, carboxylation of vitamin K–dependent factors is inhibited, resulting in nonfunctional coagulation factors. As the number of functional factors declines, hemorrhage ensues. The functional forms of prothrombin and factors VII, IX, and X disappear at a rate relative to their half-lives. Synthesis of functional factors remains inhibited until the warfarin is metabolized and cleared from the body. The duration of antagonism depends on the toxin's half-life, from several days to several weeks following ingestion of a rodenticide.

Decreased levels of vitamin K–dependent factors are manifested by abnormalities in both the PT and the APTT, since both sides of the coagulation pathway are affected. Initially the rapid disappearance of factor VII may cause prolongation of only the PT for a short period in an asymptomatic patient. However, by the time clinical bleeding becomes evident, the APTT is also prolonged, secondary to depletion of factors IX and X and prothrombin. The platelet count, fibrinogen concentration, and FDP levels usually remain normal. However, massive bleeding may reduce the platelet count to <100,000/µL, and bleeding into a body cavity may result in increased FDP levels. Correction of the coagulopathy is accomplished by administration of vitamin K_1. If bleeding is severe, transfusion of plasma will supply functional clotting factors more quickly. All of the vitamin K–dependent factors are very stable in vitro, so plasma frozen for as long as 5 years will still be effective in treatment.

Liver Disease

As most of the coagulation factors are produced in the liver, it is logical that fewer factors are produced when liver failure occurs. Generally factor depletion occurs only in very severe liver disease and is not a sensitive indicator of liver damage. In severe liver disease, multiple factors are decreased so both the PT and the APTT are prolonged. Usually other signs of liver disease such as jaundice and decreased serum albumin levels also are present.

Disseminated Intravascular Coagulation (DIC)

In patients with DIC, the coagulation mechanism in the blood is inappropriately activated (see Chapter 51). The presence of obstructing thrombi in the microcirculation stimulates endothelial cells to secrete t-PA, which initiates fibrinolysis and results in the dissolution of fibrin thrombi (Figure). Fibrin dissolution results in the formation of FDPs that enter the blood. The combination of the anticoagulant effect of the FDPs, the thrombocytopenia, and the consumption of clotting factors during thrombus formation produces hemorrhage as the primary clinical manifestation of DIC.

Formation of microthrombi throughout the vascular system can occur secondary to a variety of events, including malignancy, endotoxin exposure, infections, acute intravascular hemolysis, pancreatitis, parasite migration, heatstroke, burns, shock, and trauma. When AT III is consumed, further thrombosis is likely. Although DIC is not a primary event, if left unchecked it often results in the death of the animal, owing to the combination of thrombosis and hemorrhage within vital organs.

Acute DIC is typically characterized by thrombocytopenia; prolonged ACT, APTT, and PT; decreased fibrinogen concentration; elevated FDP levels (>40 µg/mL); and decreased AT III levels. Red cells may become fragmented when passing through thrombi in the microcirculation, resulting in the formation of schistocytes.

Chronic DIC often is more difficult to recognize because compensation by the liver and marrow in coagulation factor and platelet production can result in normalization of some of the coagulation screening parameters. Horses with DIC usually have normal fibrinogen levels.

There are many different patterns of laboratory findings, especially for chronic DIC. This should not be a surprise given an understanding that the amount of fibrinogen and number of platelets in the circulation represent a balance between the rate of synthesis and rate of consumption or destruction, and therefore are dependent on the ability of an individual's liver or marrow to respond and compensate for the depletion of factors or platelets.

Treatment for DIC should be centered on removing the underlying cause, and providing intravenous fluids to maintain blood volume and organ perfusion. Clotting factors and AT III can be replaced with transfusion of fresh-frozen plasma. Heparin is often administered to prevent further microthrombi. If the patient is bleeding, heparin should not be given unless clotting factors are replaced.

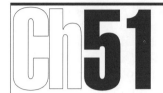
A   Arterial Thrombosis

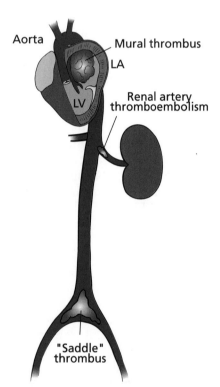

Aorta

Mural thrombus

LA

Renal artery
thromboembolism

LV

"Saddle"
thrombus

Cardiomyopathy in the cat

B   Venous Thrombosis

Vein

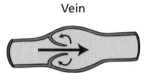

1. Stasis in valve pocket results in thrombin generation

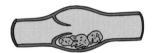

2. Platelet aggregation and fibrin formation

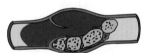

3. Blockage of venous flow with resultant retrograde extension

*T*hrombosis is an abnormality of the hemostatic mechanism in which a clot forms within the vasculature and impedes the flow of blood. Thrombi can form in arteries, veins, the heart, or the microcirculation, as in DIC (*see* Chapter 50). If a thrombus moves through the circulation and later becomes trapped at a distant site, it is called an *embolus*. Causes are varied, but thrombosis can result from an imbalance between the anticoagulant and procoagulant mechanisms.

Causes of Hypercoagulable State

Stagnant, turbulent, or misdirected blood flow allows activated platelets and coagulation factors to accumulate and initiate coagulation instead of being carried away. Abnormalities in the endothelium caused by vasculitis, laminitis in horses, or intravenous catheters, allow TF and other activators to be expressed. Conditions such as acute intravascular hemolysis, hyperadrenolcorticism, diabetes mellitus, hypercholesterolemia and deficiencies of circulating anticoagulants increase the risk of thrombosis. In patients with hepatic failure, activated coagulation factors are not removed, increasing the risk of thrombosis.

AT III Deficiency

Humans with a congenital deficiency of AT III are likely to experience repeated thrombotic events. Dogs and other animals with certain types of kidney disease such as glomerulonephritis and renal amyloidosis may lose AT III through the glomerulus. The clinical signs associated with renal protein loss are collectively called *nephrotic syndrome*, which is characterized by proteinuria, hypoalbuminemia, hyperlipidemia, and edema. Albumin is the first protein to be lost because of its small size. AT III is approximately the same size as albumin so it tends to be lost at the same time. This results in the formation of thromboemboli, especially in the lungs, but occasionally in other sites such as the portal veins and renal, femoral, or mesenteric arteries, with devastating consequences. AT III also may be consumed in patients with DIC. In humans with DIC, the degree of abnormal AT III concentration correlates inversely with survival rate.

Cardiovascular Abnormalities

Cats with cardiomyopathy often have greatly dilated atria, which generate stagnant and turbulent blood flow (**Part A**). If a clot forms, it may remain in the heart or be swept into the arterial circulation where it may become trapped where the aorta divides to supply blood to the rear legs and tail. The result is acute severe pain and posterior paralysis. Quickly the limbs become cold, and femoral pulses are absent.

Dogs with dirofilariasis (heartworms) are likely to develop pulmonary embolism because of the damaged endothelium and impaired blood flow caused by worms in the right side of the heart and pulmonary arteries. A similar problem may be seen in the mesenteric vessels of horses infected with *Strongylus* worms.

Blood vessels can be damaged in any traumatic event, whether an injury or surgical intervention. If the patient or the traumatized area such as a fracture is immobile, the risk of thrombosis increases.

Vasculitis causes activation of platelets and coagulation factors. The virus that causes feline infectious peritonitis initiates an immune response during which immune complexes damage vascular endothelium. Hemangiosarcoma with many abnormal endothelial surfaces can cause either local or disseminated intravascular coagulation that starts with thrombi in the microcirculation of the tumor itself (*see* Chapter 50).

Types of Thrombi

The composition of the thrombus varies, depending on whether it forms in an artery with high pressure and rapid blood flow, or in a vein with lower pressure (**Part B**). Arterial thrombosis is usually caused by damaged endothelium. For example, coronary thrombosis causes a "heart attack" in a human with atherosclerosis, or a thrombus may form in the heart of a dog with cardiac valvular disease. The interaction between platelets and subendothelium results in pale thrombi rich in platelets and fibrin strands with relatively few red cells.

Venous thrombi often are initiated by stasis of blood flow even with a normal vessel wall. It is suspected that the endothelium is damaged subsequently by hypoxia, resulting in platelet activation. The resulting thrombus tends to contain many red cells that become trapped as they pass through the area. Thus, venous thrombi resemble the clots seen in test tubes after blood is drawn. They sometimes are called *red thrombi* and commonly occlude the veins. Most venous thrombi also have a white platelet-rich head and a long red tail dangling downstream. Bits of these clots are detached easily and travel to the lungs (pulmonary embolism). If large emboli obstruct major pulmonary arteries, death may follow because of right ventricular failure secondary to decreased pulmonary blood flow. The consequences of arterial emboli may be minor as with small infarcts found incidentally at surgery or severe as with obstructed renal arteries causing renal shutdown. Emboli may also consist of fat, air, or even a foreign body that has invaded the circulation. Embolic material infected with microorganisms is called a *septic embolus* and may disseminate an infection.

Diagnosis of thromboembolic disease can be difficult. Imaging techniques such as ultrasonography or nuclear scans may be useful. Sometimes the problem is suspected because of the known predisposition of some underlying diseases. Heparin treatment might be given prophylactically in some situations of very high risk. Once a thrombus has formed, treatment is more difficult and drugs such as streptokinase, or tPA might be needed (*see* Chapter 44). Fortunately minor thromboembolic episodes often resolve spontaneously, and collateral circulation provides blood flow peripheral to the thrombus until the occluded vessel becomes patent again.

Ch52 Hematopoietic Malignancy

A **Action of Oncogenes**

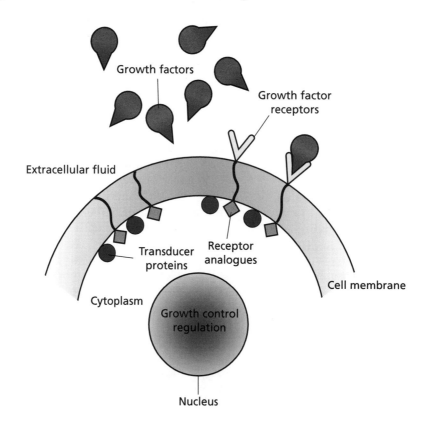

Growth factors

Growth factor receptors

Extracellular fluid

Transducer proteins

Receptor analogues

Cell membrane

Cytoplasm

Growth control regulation

Nucleus

B **Chromosomal Translocation**

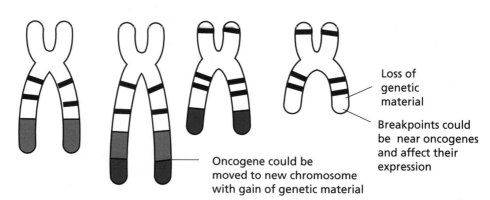

Loss of genetic material

Breakpoints could be near oncogenes and affect their expression

Oncogene could be moved to new chromosome with gain of genetic material

Loss or gain of genetic material
Loss of material from one chromosome and added to another.

Leukemias and lymphomas are cancers caused by unregulated, self-perpetuating, and abnormal proliferation of hematopoietic cells (*see* Chapters 53–55).

Knowledge of leukemia can be traced back to the mid-1800s, shortly after the microscope was first utilized to examine tissues. Hematopoietic malignancies kill patients, not necessarily because the cells divide too rapidly, but because they never stop dividing. Eventually production of normal hematopoietic cells is suppressed, and other tissues are invaded and damaged, causing signs of illness and impaired organ function.

Most malignancies result from the transformation and proliferation of a single cell (clonal expansion theory). An acquired chromosomal derangement—either translocation, deletion, or amplification—causes arrest at some stage of maturation of a hematopoietic precursor. When the defect affects very early stem cells, all hematopoietic cell lines are affected. Such stem cell disorders include myelogenous leukemias and myelodysplasia (*see* Chapters 54 and 55). Although no malignant cells may be seen in patients with myelodysplasia, cytogenetic studies of humans with these disorders usually show specific chromosomal changes associated with malignancy. If a chromosomal change occurs farther along the maturation pathway, malignancies with characteristics of specific myeloid or lymphoid cell lines occur.

Leukemia originates in the bone marrow and is not one, but a whole group of diseases. They are classified as lymphoid or nonlymphoid (myeloid), and acute, or chronic. These classifications have treatment and prognostic implications.

Etiology and Epidemiology

In animals, leukemia and lymphoma occur most frequently in cats, dogs, and humans. Although the causes of cancer are complex and only partly understood, molecular techniques are leading to improvements in our knowledge. Whenever DNA is damaged beyond the ability for the cell to repair it, but not enough to kill the cell, the chance for transformation is present. Several insults are often necessary to cause a cancer cell to emerge. Some causes are viruses, radiation, carcinogens, and aberrations of the immune system.

Oncogenes and Suppressor Genes

An important discovery in the mechanisms of leukemogenesis came with the observation that changes in the structure or location of certain normal cellular genes caused cells to transform into tumor cells. These genes, called *oncogenes* (e.g., *src, ras, abl*) were first identified in association with retroviruses causing malignancies in animals. These viruses insert next to an oncogene, either activating it directly or interfering with an inhibitor. In other cases, viruses pick up normal host cellular proto-oncogenes, which normally serve as growth regulatory genes. Oncogenes function as growth factors, growth factor receptors, transducers of signals from the cytoplasm to the nucleus, and tyrosine kinases that induce cell division (**Part A**). In the nucleus, oncogenes act as transcription factors that bind to DNA and regulate messenger RNA synthesis. When they become activated inappropriately, these genes direct cells to divide uncontrollably.

Oncogenes can be turned on by other mechanisms to cause malignancies of nonviral origin. The action of 1 oncogene may not be sufficient to cause malignancy by itself. Genetic translocations might place an oncogene next to a growth factor gene, or cause other chromosomal damage or mutation (**Part B**). This same chromosomal abnormality can be seen in all of the tumor cells in an individual, and in others with the same type of malignancy.

Other genes such as *p53* act to suppress transformation. Detections or mutations of the *p53* gene greatly increase the risk of malignancy.

Oncogenic Viruses

Viruses are known to cause leukemia in cats, cattle, mice, poultry, fish, and primates, including humans. Viruses were first suspected to be oncogenic when sarcomas in chickens were passed from one to another by filtered extracts of tumor tissue. The Rous sarcoma virus was later identified as an RNA virus of the retrovirus family. The name *retrovirus* comes from *reverse transcriptase*, an enzyme that enables transcription of a DNA copy of the virus, which is then integrated into the genome of the host. For a virus to cause cancer, it must be a DNA virus such as the herpesvirus that causes Marek's disease (a form of lymphoma) in poultry, or it must have a DNA phase, as do retroviruses. Murine leukemias caused by retroviruses have been studied extensively as models of viral oncogenesis. These viruses are passed genetically from mother to offspring and result in malignancy in a high percentage of susceptible strains. The discovery of FeLV resulted in identification of the first malignancy caused by a virus in an outbred mammalian species, and led to a search for human cancer viruses. Bovine leukemia virus is an important cause of lymphoma in cattle. In humans, a retrovirus, human T-cell lymphotropic virus type 1 (HTLV-1), can cause lymphoma, and DNA viruses have been associated with lymphoma (herpesvirus) and liver cancer (hepadnovirus).

Radiation, Chemical Carcinogens, and Genetic Predisposition

Radiation causes damage to DNA which may result in leukemia in humans or animals. Chemicals also can cause leukemia. Benzene and alkylating agents used for cancer chemotherapy are the most notorious, but cases in humans have been linked to drugs such as phenylbutazone and chloramphenicol. Genetic susceptibility to leukemia and lymphoma exists in humans and animals. Boxer dogs and possibly golden retrievers have a higher incidence than other breeds. People with certain genetic immunodeficiency diseases are at increased risk of developing malignancy.

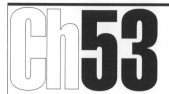 **Lymphoma**

Comparison Between Species

	Dogs	Cats	Cattle	Horse
Causes	Unknown	FeLV	BoLV in adults	Unknown
Age	Middle – old age	Any age	Young – middle age	Middle age
Most common presentation	Generalized lymphadenopathy	Alimentary or mediastinal	Juvenile lymphadenopathy marrow Adolescent mediastinal Adult lymphadenopathy	Lymphadenopathy Visceral Skin
Histology	Most high grade*	Most high grade	High grade	Low to high grade

* High-grade lymphoma is usually a lymphoblastic or immunoblastic phenotype.
Low-grade is also called well-differentiated lymphocytic lymphoma.

Lymphoma is the most common hematopoietic tumor of dogs and cats and is relatively common in cattle, horses, pigs, and chickens. Synonyms include lymphosarcoma, malignant lymphoma, and non-Hodgkin's lymphoma; in chickens, the term *leukosis* is used sometimes. Lymphoma is a malignant solid tumor of monoclonal lymphoid origin, but must be considered as a systemic disease. When treated with chemotherapy, lymphoma tends to be among the most responsive of all malignancies.

Within an individual patient, 1 subset of lymphocytes becomes malignant (**Figure**). The behavior and prognosis of the various forms differ. Well-differentiated lymphocytic (low-grade) lymphoma is rare and usually slowly progressive. Poorly differentiated, diffuse lymphoblastic and immunoblastic (both high-grade) lymphomas are more common and rapidly progressive. In general, B-cell (most commonly immunoblastic) lymphoma has a better prognosis for response to treatment and survival than does T-cell (usually lymphoblastic) lymphoma. Special techniques beyond histological examination are required for identification of B-cell, T-cell, or other cell-surface markers. Although lymphoid organs are most involved, the tumors can invade almost any tissue in the body and may seem to arise simultaneously from several sites.

In Dogs

The incidence of lymphoma in dogs is 13–14 cases/100,000 dogs/year, by far the most common hematopoietic tumor. Affected dogs are most often middle-aged or older, and breeds such as boxers and golden retrievers appear to be at increased risk. Life expectancy after diagnosis averages about 2 months, but with chemotherapy the median survival time is about 1 year.

The most common presentation is diffuse lymphadenopathy. Most dogs do not have signs of illness at the time of diagnosis, but later become progressively debilitated as the tumor invades vital organs. About 15%–20%, usually those with T-cell lymphoma, have hypercalcemia (pseudohyperparathyroidism) at the time of diagnosis. This is caused by elaboration of a parathyroid-like hormone by the lymphoblasts and causes signs of polydipsia, polyuria, and renal damage. If the bone marrow is invaded, neutropenia, thrombocytopenia, and anemia add to the morbidity and make treatment more difficult (*see* Chapter 54).

In Cats

At one time the incidence of feline lymphoma was estimated at 200 cases/100,000 cats/year, but this is decreasing as testing and vaccination have made FeLV less common. The virus is spread in a contagious manner and kittens are most susceptible to infection. The virus is spread only by direct exposure to blood, saliva or respiratory secretions of an infected cat. Most cats infected with FeLV never develop leukemia or lymphoma, but die of anemia or infectious diseases secondary to FeLV-induced immunosuppression. Most viremic cats remain persistently infected, but a few develop a successful immune response and are no longer viremic.

The average age of occurrence of lymphoma is 3 years for viremic and 7 years for nonviremic cats.

In contrast to dogs, most feline lymphoma involves visceral organs rather than peripheral lymph nodes. The most common sites of involvement are the gastrointestinal (alimentary) tract and anterior mediastinum. Other frequently affected sites are the kidneys, liver, spleen, epidural space (especially in the lumbar region), nose, eyes, and skin. Alimentary lymphoma is usually of B-cell origin, is FeLV negative, and is found in old cats, whereas mediastinal lymphoma is usually of T-cell origin, is viremic, and is seen in younger cats. Treatment is similar for cats and dogs. Cats are somewhat more difficult to treat since visceral involvement increases the risk of morbidity from the disease and the treatment.

In Cattle

Bovine lymphoma is a B-cell malignancy caused by a retrovirus, bovine leukemia virus (BoLV). Antibody to BoLV is found in approximately 60% of all dairy herds in the United States. The virus appears to be spread from the cow to the calf through the milk, possibly in leukocytes. The virus also may be spread by infected blood transferred through needles or contaminated gloves used for rectal examinations.

Some cattle develop persistent lymphocytosis when infected with BoLV, but this may regress spontaneously or lymphoma may develop later.

Bovine lymphoma occurs as juvenile, an adolescent, and adult forms only the adult form is caused by BoLV. The juvenile form occurs up to the age of 6 months and is characterized by lymphadenopathy, sometimes with anemia and malignant cells in the marrow and the blood. The adolecent form occurs at ages 6–18 months and is primarily associated with a mediastinal mass. The adult form, usually develops between ages 5 and 8 years and most often involves lymph nodes.

In Humans

Human non-Hodgkin's lymphomas have been well characterized by cell-surface markers and lymphocytic subgroups. Lymphoma is a heterogeneous disease morphologically and immunologically.

Hodgkin's disease is classified as a lymphoma because it usually arises in lymph nodes with characteristic giant cells known as Reed-Sternberg cells. Hodgkin's disease has not been found in animals.

In Other Species

Lymphoma is known to occur in most mammalian species. It is diagnosed occasionally in horses, often with visceral or cutaneous involvement. As ferrets have become popular as pets, lymphoma has been diagnosed frequently, both as an acute disease of young animals and as a chronic disease of older animals.

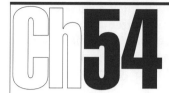

Acute Leukemia

A   Comparison of Acute and Chronic Leukemia in Dogs and Cats

	Acute	Chronic
Age	All ages	Older age
Clinical onset	Sudden	Indolent
Leukemic cells	Immature	Mature
Anemia, thrombocytopenia	Prominent	Mild or absent
WBC count	Variable	Increased

B   Classifications of Acute Leukemias

Lymphoid – ALL
    T- or B-cell origin or unclassified
    Subtypes of T-cell ALL exist

Nonlymphoid – AML
    Classification (French, American, British)
        M_1 – Myeloblastic without maturation
        M_2 – Myeloblastic with some maturation
        M_3 – Promyelocytic
        M_4 – Myelomonocytic
        M_5 – Monocytic
        M_6 – Erythroleukemia
        M_7 – Acute megakaroblastic leukemia

Leukemias are broadly classified as acute or chronic, and as lymphoid or nonlymphoid (myelogenous). Acute leukemia, is characterized by infiltration (>30% of nucleated cells) and often replacement of the marrow by blasts that proliferate but do not mature or function in any useful way. Any hematopoietic cell line can be involved. Progression of the disease is rapid, with death occurring within days to weeks after the onset of clinical disease if treatment is not given or is unsuccessful. Chronic leukemias also are characterized by some infiltration of the marrow, but usually to a lesser extent, with preservation of normal hematopoiesis until late in the course of the disease (**Part A**). In chronic leukemia, the malignant cells continue to mature, but simply fail to stop proliferating in the absence of growth factors.

Clinical signs of acute leukemia of any cell type are referable to bone marrow infiltration resulting in nonregenerative anemia, granulocytopenia with infections, and thrombocytopenia with bleeding. If the bone marrow is the principal site of involvement, the disease is classified as leukemia regardless of the presence or absence of circulating blasts. Although leukemia often is associated with large numbers of circulating blasts, the typical blood cell count in a leukemic patient is often normal or low. Severe leukocytosis with blasts is the exception rather than the rule. In acute leukemia the bone marrow usually is packed with blasts at the time of diagnosis, although myelodysplastic ("preleukemic") syndromes exist with abnormal hematopoiesis, but without diagnostic numbers of blasts present. Classification of the subtypes of acute leukemia by morphological description of the blasts is difficult to impossible in many cases. Use of cell-surface markers, cytochemistry, and more recently in humans, chromosomal markers has allowed more accurate classification. The identification of acute lymphoblastic leukemia (ALL) has clinical significance, as dogs and cats with ALL have about a 25% chance of remission when treated with chemotherapy. With currently available drug protocols, the response rate of acute myelogenous leukemia (AML) is close to zero.

ALL

In ALL, the marrow is infiltrated with variable numbers of circulating lymphoblasts. Splenomegaly and sometimes hepatomegaly may be present, but other tumor masses are typically absent. If the primary clinical signs are referable to the marrow, the disease is called *ALL* even though some organomegaly is present. If the primary presentation is because of lymphadenopathy or dyspnea from a mediastinal mass, the disease is called *lymphoma* even if blasts are circulating in the blood, or if a bone marrow study shows malignant infiltration. Lymphoma with involvement of the marrow is classified as stage V, which is the highest stage with the worst prognosis. The distinction between stage V lymphoma and ALL with organomegaly is somewhat artificial since the 2 diseases overlap, and the difference is primarily geographical.

Subgroups of ALL comparable to various subsets of lymphocytes are recognized in humans. The lack of readily available, species-specific reagents interferes with classification beyond B- and T-cell origin in dogs and cats. Not only is leukemia composed of multiple diseases, but also ALL is a heterogeneous disorder with variability in behavior.

AML

The acute nonlymphocytic leukemias include granulocytic, monocytic, erythroid, or megakaryocytic elements and are jointly referred to as *AML*. The term *myeloproliferative disease* is sometimes used to include both acute and chronic myelogenous leukemias, myelodysplasia, and myelofibrosis. In adult humans, AML is the most common form of acute leukemia. AML occurs in dogs and cats and is rare in other species except for laboratory rodents.

Depending on which cell line is predominant, AML is subclassified as myeloblastic, promyelocytic, myelomonocytic, monocytic, erythroleukemia, or megakaryocytic. A classification used for AML is given in **Part B**. The clinical presentation is identical to that of ALL. Abnormal cells may be present in high numbers in the blood or be totally absent. The bone marrow contains from 30% to almost 100% blasts. The various blasts have some distinguishing morphological features that help in classification of the type of leukemia, but sometimes the blasts are so undifferentiated that morphological classification beyond that of acute leukemia may be impossible.

Within AML, myeloblastic leukemia may be undifferentiated or show some signs of differentiation toward granulocytic lineage. Promyelocytic leukemia is characterized by a marrow filled with promyelocytes, large cells with pink primary granules. Myelomonocytic leukemia shows characteristics of both granulocytes and monocytes, suggesting a transformation event before these 2 cells diverged in their maturation pathway. In monocytic leukemia, the marrow is filled with monoblasts despite the name, which might imply that mature monocytes are involved. Erythroleukemia is characterized by replacement of the marrow with immature nonfunctional red cell precursors, resulting in severe *nonregenerative* anemia with reticulocytopenia. Nucleated red cells, primarily metarubricytes, but some rubricytes, prorubricytes, and even rubriblasts may be present in the blood as well as the marrow. Megaloblastic changes, asynchronous maturation of the nucleus and cytoplasm, and skipped mitoses resulting in giant immature forms of erythroid and sometimes granulocytic cells may be seen. Acute megakaryocytic leukemia is characterized by immature and abnormal megakaryocytes in the marrow, and usually thrombocytopenia in the blood.

Techniques such as cytochemical staining, assays to determine the presence or absence of certain cell membrane antigens, and cytogenetic studies are used to differentiate subtypes of acute leukemia. The most important point is that all acute leukemias, regardless of cell type, are characterized clinically by neutropenia, anemia, and thrombocytopenia, caused by a factor elaborated by the malignant blasts that suppresses normal hematopoiesis.

Ch55 Chronic Leukemia

A Classification of Chronic Leukemias

Lymphoid – Chronic lymphocytic leukemia (CLL)
Granulocytic – Chronic Myelogenous (granulocytic) leukemia (CML)
Erythroid – Polycythemia rubra vera
Megakaryocytic – Essential thrombocythemia
Myelodysplasia – Preleukemia
Myelofibrosis – Malignancy?

B Typical Hemograms for CLL, CML, P Vera, and Essential Thrombocythemia in a Dog (see reference ranges in Chapter 58)

	CLL	CML	P vera	Thrombocytosis
Hct (%)	35	35	70	25
RBC indices	Normal	Normal	Normal	Normal
WBC (ml)	75,000	75,000	20,000	5000
Neutophils (ml)	9000	39,000	15,000	3000
Bands (ml)	0	12,000	1000	0
Metamyelocytes (ml)	0	15,000	0	0
Myelocytes (ml)	0	5000	0	0
Lymphocytes (ml)	65,000	1000	1000	1000
Monocytes (ml)	1000	1000	1000	1000
Eosinophils (ml)	0	2000	2000	0
Platelet count (ml)	180,000	180,000	180,000	1,500,000

Chronic Lymphocytic Leukemia (CLL)

Chronic leukemias are characterized by some infiltration of the marrow, but the malignant cells are more likely to mature partially or completely and retain some or all of their function. Progression is slow, and survival may be for months to years, sometimes with minimal or no treatment. The classification used for chronic leukemias and the typical changes in hemograms are shown in **Parts A** and **B**.

Chronic Lymphocytic Leukemia (CLL)

CLL primarily affects older dogs and humans and is characterized by increased numbers of mature, lymphocytes, usually of B-cell origin, that look normal but function abnormally. These cells have difficulty passing through the endothelium of vessels and accumulate in the blood. Many cases are found incidentally when a blood cell count is done for some other reason. Splenomegaly sometimes with mild lymphadenopathy is often present, usually without anemia, neutropenia, or thrombocytopenia because the marrow retains normal hematopoietic precursors. It is important to differentiate this disease from ALL as the prognosis is better and the progression slower with CLL. The diagnosis is one of excluding other causes of lymphocytosis. If the lymphocytosis is mild, between 10,000 and 20,000 cells/μL, and no other cause is evident, a diagnosis of CLL is suspected, but cell counts may have to be monitored over time to see if the count continues to rise. Fortunately this delay does not harm the patient as early treatment does not change the overall survival rate. Treatment usually is instituted when lymphocyte counts reach 50,000/μL or other cytopenias occur. Because the CLL cells are slow to divide, but survive for long periods, response to treatment may take several weeks.

Chronic Myelogenous Leukemia (CML)

CML is characterized by a proliferation of granulocytes that maintain some normal function and morphology. A characteristic chromosomal translocation, called *Philadelphia chromosome,* is present in affected humans, but not in animals. This translocation is present in all of the myeloid precursors in the marrow, suggesting that transformation occurred at the stem cell level. This disease is seen rarely in animals, with most of the reported cases occurring in dogs. Clinically CML is characterized by marked neutrophilia and a significant left shift. The term *leukemoid reaction* is used to describe a neutrophilia and left shift in situations of pyogenic inflammation so severe that the CBC resembles that seen with CML. Animals with leukemoid reactions usually are febrile and quite ill, and the WBC count drops after a few days of successful treatment. In contrast, CML causes minimal morbidity initially, but the disease progresses after 2–3 years to "blast crisis," characterized by an outpouring of blasts refractory to chemotherapy.

Polycythemia Rubra Vera (P vera)

This disease of humans, dogs, and cats is characterized by an autonomous overproduction of functional, mature red cells (*see* also Chapter 28). The total red cell mass is increased, resulting in sludging of the blood causing congestive heart failure and decreased oxygenation of the brain. The marrow shows increased erythroid production, with normal maturation. The malignant clone of erythroid cells proliferates without regard for the normal negative feedback inhibition of decreased erythropoietin. P vera is the red cell equivalent of CML or CLL. Treatment of P vera involves removal of excessive red cells by phlebotomy until the Hct approaches normal. Most cases in humans, dogs, and cats can be controlled by chemotherapy for months to years.

Essential Thrombocytosis

Platelets can be produced autonomously in excessive numbers, usually >1,000,000/μL in essential thrombocytosis, which is a very rare disease. The FeLV-positive cat is most likely to be victimized. Although thrombotic or hemorrhagic complications have occurred in humans, these problems have not occurred in affected cats.

Myelodysplasia (Myelodysplastic Syndrome, MDS) and Myelofibrosis

Myelodysplasia is associated with faulty maturation and cell division involving the granulocyte, erythrocyte, and megakaryocyte series, either singly or more often, in combination. The bone marrow is usually normocellular or hypercellular despite peripheral cytopenias (ineffective hematopoiesis). Myelodysplasia is considered to be a stage in the evolution of AML and is sometimes referred to as *preleukemia*. In humans, specific chromosomal abnormalities imply that myelodysplasia is a clonal disorder even though no neoplastic cells are present initially.

A refractory anemia is the most common finding in the blood. Thrombocytopenia, leukopenia, or both also may occur. Frequent findings are increased nucleated RBC counts without reticulocytosis, and large bizarre platelets. Characteristic findings in erythroid precursors in the marrow include asynchronous maturation in which the cytoplasm of the cell matures more quickly than the nucleus. Maturation arrest of granulocyte precursors is characterized by the presence of giant band neutrophils, abnormal granulation, or abnormal nuclei. Megakaryoctes may have abnormal morphology. Treatment of MDS is primarily supportive with transfusions given as needed. Chemotherapy has not proved to be beneficial.

Myelofibrosis has been included in the myeloproliferative diseases on the basis that it may represent a malignant proliferation of fibroblasts filling the marrow and inhibiting hematopoiesis. Probably more likely, it represents an "end-stage" marrow, analogous to cirrhosis of the liver.

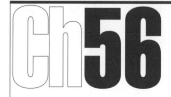

Plasma Cell Neoplasms

A   Pathogenesis of Myeloma

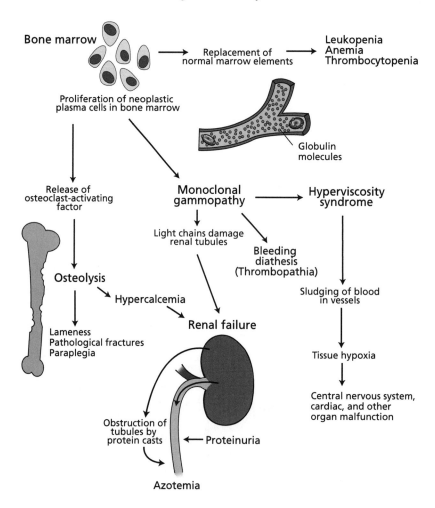

Bone marrow → Replacement of normal marrow elements → Leukopenia, Anemia, Thrombocytopenia

Proliferation of neoplastic plasma cells in bone marrow

Globulin molecules

Release of osteoclast-activating factor

Monoclonal gammopathy → Hyperviscosity syndrome

Light chains damage renal tubules

Bleeding diathesis (Thrombopathia)

Osteolysis

Hypercalcemia

Sludging of blood in vessels

Renal failure

Lameness
Pathological fractures
Paraplegia

Tissue hypoxia

Central nervous system, cardiac, and other organ malfunction

Obstruction of tubules by protein casts ← Proteinuria

Azotemia

B   Electrophoresis of Canine Serum

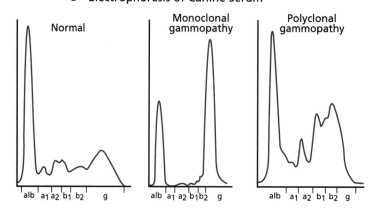

Normal

Monoclonal gammopathy

Polyclonal gammopathy

alb a₁ a₂ b₁ b₂ g

Myeloma (center) is associated with a monoclonal spike on electrphoresis. Decreased levels of other globulin subclasses and hypoalbuminemia may occur as well. Polyclonal gammopathy (right) encountered in chronic infections is characterized by elevated levels of all subclasses of globulins.

Since plasma cells are differentiated B cells, the malignancies of plasma cells can be grouped with the lymphoproliferative malignancies.

Myeloma

Myeloma has also been referred to as *plasma cell myeloma* or *multiple myeloma*. Myeloma has been described in dogs, horses, cows, pigs, mice, rabbits, cats, and humans. The disease usually begins in the marrow and invades and lyses bone to produce punched-out, well-circumscribed, lytic lesions that are diffuse in flat bones and sometimes in long bones (**Part A**). The disease can be indicated by the presence of bone pain or pathological fracture. If vertebrae are involved, paraplegia may occur. Hypercalcemia and secondary renal failure can occur if bone lysis is extensive. The tumor cells are primarily immature plasma cells that usually secrete immunoglobulin.

Serum protein electrophoresis (SPEP) may identify a narrow monoclonal spike in the β or γ region. Once the monoclonal gammopathy is recognized, the specific class of abnormal immunoglobulin can be identified by immunoelectrophoresis. The monoclonal immunoglobulin is sometimes referred to as the *paraprotein* or *M component* (**Part B**). Because all of these molecules are synthesized by progeny of a single lymphoid cell, they are monoclonal, meaning they are chemically identical, travel together, and appear as a tight band on electrophoresis. In normal individuals without myeloma, stimulation of the immune system by infection or other antigen leads to increased antibody production resulting in a broad-based elevation in the γ region of the SPEP, designated accordingly as a polyclonal gammopathy.

Myelomas usually secrete IgG or IgA and are the most common cause of monoclonal gammopathy. Other less common causes include B-cell lymphomas, CLL, and occasionally some infections such as ehrlichiosis in dogs.

Free light chains, also known as *Bence Jones proteins,* are found frequently in the urine of patients with myeloma. The detection of Bence Jones proteins by urine protein electrophoresis is important because of the high rate of renal failure associated with their presence. The "dipsticks" employed for rapid urine screening for albuminuria do not register free light chain as a protein because of its positive charge.

Anemia, bleeding tendencies, or recurring infections are other reasons for presentation. Cytopenias can result from infiltration of the marrow with immature plasma cells. Bleeding can result from thrombocytopenia or from abnormal platelet function caused by coating of the platelets with immunoglobulin, which interferes with aggregation. The most common sites of bleeding are the nose and the gingiva. The increased risk of infections is related to the fact that production of functional immunoglobulins is suppressed by the paraprotein. Neutropenia might also occur if the marrow is heavily infiltrated by plasma cells.

Myeloma responds relatively well to chemotherapy, and survival times beyond a year are relatively common.

Bone pain decreases, but bone lesions are slow to heal. The risk of fractures remains for several weeks even if the response to treatment is good.

Waldenström's Macroglobulinemia and Hyperviscosity

Waldenström's macroglobulinemia, a malignancy of "plasmacytoid" B cells, is closely related to myeloma and produces high concentrations of IgM. Hyperviscosity occurs with macroglobulinemia (IgM), but also may occur with polymerized IgA. The flow characteristics of blood are determined by interactions between the red cells and the proteins of the suspending plasma. Blood viscosity increases rapidly with increasing concentrations of larger molecules of the plasma, such as IgM. Because plasma proteins serve as electrical insulators, elevated concentrations allow red cells (normally negatively charged) to come closer to each other and form weak agglutinates, a phenomenon known as *rouleau formation*. Rouleaux appear as microscopic "stacks of coins" in blood smears. Whenever rouleaux are seen on a blood smear, the serum proteins should be evaluated. Rouleaux are normal in horses, and to a lesser extent in cats.

Hyperviscosity, whether caused by high Hct or hyperproteinemia, causes serious pathophysiological changes: neurological signs from poor oxygenation of the brain, and peripheral vascular resistance, leading to hypertension and heart failure. Dilated retinal vessels may be visible on examination of the eye. Viscosity, as evaluated by a viscometer, is the serum viscosity relative to water (normally 1–2). A relative serum viscosity ≥4 represents an emergency. The mechanisms of clinical signs are probably sludging of blood in small vessels. The blood volume is increased in many patients with hyperviscosity syndrome because of increased osmotic pressure in the vessels. Sometimes hyperproteinemia can be detected on a routine blood smear because of the presence of a hazy blue background.

The treatment of hyperviscosity syndrome must be directed first toward rapid reduction of the viscosity. This is accomplished by removal of plasma manually or by plasmapheresis. Plasma is replaced partly by normal plasma and partly by crystalloid. This procedure can be repeated periodically as needed. Depending on how fast the abnormal globulin is replaced, chemotherapy may be needed.

Extramedullary Plasma Cell Tumors

A plasma cell tumor that affects soft tissue instead of bone or bone marrow is referred to as an *extramedullary plasmacytoma*. These tumors are relatively common in dogs. Most are benign, but a few metastasize and some produce immunoglobulin. The most frequent sites are skin and mucocutaneous junctions, and less commonly the gastrointestinal tract.

Other Hematopoietic Malignancies

Comparison Between Systemic and Malignant Histiocytosis

	Signalment	Clinical Course	History	Location of Lesions	Histiopathology
SH	Young – middle-aged Primarily males Primarily Bernese mountain dog	Chronic intermittent	Skin nodules May have no systemic signs	Primarily skin/ lymph nodes Multiple nodules Lymphadenopathy Sometimes ocular lesions	Histiocytic infiltration Morphology near normal
MH	Middle-aged – to old Primarily males Primarily Bernese mountain dog Golden and flat coated retrievers and Rottweilers may be predisposed as well Has been reportred in cats	Rapidly fatal	Dyspnea Weight loss Weakness	Lung, spleen Bone marrow Neurological involvement Anemia common Splenomegaly common Skin and eyes rarely involved	Large atypical histiocytes High mitotic index Giant cells present Erythrophagocytosis May need immuno- histochemistry to differentiate from lymphoma or other poorly differentiated neoplasms

SH = systemic histiocytosis
MH = malignant histiocyctosis

Mast Cell Tumors

Mast cell tumors are included with the hematopoietic malignancies because the precursors of the mast cell probably originate in the marrow even though they mature in the connective tissue. Mast cell tumors are quite common in dogs, fairly common in cats, and rare in other species.

Canine Mast Cell Tumors

In dogs, mast cell tumors most commonly occur as skin tumors. Those that are well differentiated are usually curable by wide and deep excision. Those of intermediate differentiation are most common and have a high rate of local recurrence. Poorly differentiated mast cell tumors are likely to spread to regional lymph nodes. Some become disseminated, especially in the marrow and spleen. Dogs may be euthanized because of tumor ulceration, bleeding, and secondary infection.

Mast cell granules contain histamine, heparin, platelet-activating factor, and other active substances (see Chapter 35). Release of granule contents can cause local edema and gastric ulceration secondary to increased secretion of hydrochloric acid in response to histamine. Heparin can exacerbate local bleeding. Diagnosis of superficial mast cell tumors is usually easy as mast cells are visible on cytological preparations of needle aspirates.

Feline Mast Cell Tumors

The skin is the most common site of mast cell tumors in the cat, but the tumor behaves somewhat differently. Most single tumors in cats are curable by surgery. Multiple skin masses occur more commonly, but they tend to grow slowly. The cat is more likely than the dog to have "mast cell leukemia," characterized by primary involvement of the marrow and spleen even without skin masses. The spleen may be massively enlarged, and mast cells may be present in the blood. Anemia may occur but is usually less severe than that seen in leukemias of other types. FeLV does not seem to be associated with mastocytosis. The clinical signs of disseminated mast cell tumor are similar in cats and dogs. The development of duodenal ulcers is especially dangerous because these ulcers can perforate and cause peritonitis as a terminal event.

Malignancies of Histiocytic Origin

Benign Cutaneous Histiocytomas

These tumors, which are common in young dogs, appear as well-circumscribed, raised, hairless, sometimes ulcerated skin nodules. Occasionally there are multiple nodules. The cell of origin is a dermal macrophage. Most regress spontaneously; the rest are cured with surgical excision.

Systemic Histiocytosis

The middle-aged Bernese mountain dog has a hereditary predisposition to develop systemic histiocytosis. This disease is characterized by multiple cutaneous masses, some of which may be ulcerated. Lesions come and go over weeks to months and sometimes spread to regional lymph nodes and even abdominal organs. The cells in the lesions are primarily histiocytes, and it is not clear if this is a reactive or a neoplastic proliferation (**Figure**).

Malignant Histiocytosis

This aggressive malignant proliferation of histiocytes occurs most commonly in Bernese mountain dogs, but also can be seen in other large breed dogs, especially Rottweilers, and Labrador and golden retrievers. It has been found rarely in cats. The lung is commonly involved, with the proliferation being either a solitary mass, multiple nodules, or diffuse infiltrate. The bone marrow is frequently involved, and splenomegaly is common. The resulting cytopenias sometimes cause confusion with immune-mediated hemolysis. Central nervous system involvement can cause seizures or paralysis. The malignant cells are large, bizarre histiocytic cells, sometimes with erythrophagocytosis. This disease is quite resistant to treatment, and the survival time for most affected dogs is days to weeks after diagnosis. It generally is thought that this disease is different from systemic histiocytosis, but intermediate cases appear, albeit very rarely. Malignant histiocytosis must not be confused with another soft-tissue tumor called *malignant fibrous histiocytosis,* which is closely related to fibrosarcomas and not related to these histiocytic tumors.

Transmissible Venereal Tumor (TVT)

The canine TVT is unique among neoplasms in that it actually arises from cells transmitted from an affected dog to a susceptible dog through direct, usually sexual contact. The tumor cell is probably of histiocytic origin and contains fewer chromosomes than does the normal canine genome, 58 or 59 rather than the usual 78. This same cytogenetic change is seen in all tumors examined throughout the world. When cells are transmitted, usually through coitus, tumors appear on the male or female external genitalia. Occasionally TVTs occur on the nose or mouth. These tumors are friable and frequently bleed, but metastasize only very rarely. Experimentally produced tumors regress spontaneously, but most naturally occurring tumors persist and are a source of discomfort. Fortunately they are almost 100% curable with chemotherapy, and an ongoing immune response prevents reinfection.

Reference Values
for Various Species

A   Reference Range for Hematology Parameters

	Dog	Cat	Horse	Cow	Sheep*
HCT (%)	37–55	30–45	32–48	24-46	24–50
Hb (gm/dL)	12–18	8–15	11–19	8–15	8–16
MCV (fL)	60–77	39–55	37–58	40–60	23–48
MCHC (gm/dL)	32–36	30–36	31–37	30–36	31–34
MCH (pg/dL)	19–24	13–17	13–19	11–17	—
Reticulocytes (%)	0–1	0–1	0	0	0
WBCs (10^3 /mL)	6–17	5–19	5–12	4–12	4–12
Neutrophils (mL)	3–11	2–12	3–7	0.6–4.0	0.7–6.0
Bands (10^3 /mL)	<0.3	<0.3	<0.1	<0.1	<0.1
Lymphocytes (10^3 /mL)	1–5	1–7	1–5	2–7	2–9
Monocytes (10^3 mL)	0–1.5	0–1	0–1	0–1	0–1
Eosinophils (10^3 /mL)	0–1	0–1	0–1	0–2	0–1
Total serum protein (gm/dL)	6.0–7.5	6.0–7.5	6–8	6–8	6–8
Platelets (10^3 /mL)	200–500	200–700	100–600	100–600	200–700

*Goat is similar to sheep except MCV (fL) = 15 – 30.

B   Reference Range for Coagulation Parameters

	Dog	Cat	Horse	Cow	Sheep
PT (sec)	8–9	8–10	9–12	10–20	—
APTT (sec)	12–19	12–17	42–65	30–90	34–51
Fibrinogen (mg/dL)	100–500	50–300	100–500	200–800	—
ACT (sec)	<120	<120	—	—	—
FDP (mg/mL)	<10	<10	<10	<10	—

ecause memorization of reference values for each species is not practical, it is more helpful to think in generalities. For example, 30%–50% is a normal PCV for most species. The size and number of RBCs vary among species. The smaller the RBC, the greater the number per unit of volume. Many small RBCs are more efficient in distributing oxygen to the tissues than are a few larger ones. This is related to the increased surface area–volume ratio for small cells. Sheep and goats have the smallest RBCs of the domestic species, and dogs have the largest. Ancestors of sheep and goats lived at high altitudes where their small cells were an advantage. This characteristic has remained in domestic breeds even though the need is no longer present. Rouleaux are marked in the horse.

A WBC count within the reference range for most species is 5,000–13,000/µL. Ruminants may have slightly lower counts and have more lymphocytes than neutrophils, whereas dogs, cats, and horses have primarily neutrophils. WBCs in dogs and cats respond more to adrenal corticosteroid hormone (stress) than do those of ruminants. An eosinophil count >1,000–1,500/µL is abnormal in all species. Refer to **Parts A** and **B** as abnormalities are discussed.

References

Babior B, Stossel T. *Hematology, a pathophysiological approach,* 3rd ed. New York: Churchill Livingstone, 1994. (Paperback on humans but very readable and most is appropriate for veterinary medicine)

Duncan JR, Prasse KW. *Veterinary laboratory medicine,* 3rd ed. Ames: Iowa State University Press, 1994. (Outline of veterinary hematology)

Ettinger SJ, Feldman SJ. *Textbook of veterinary internal medicine,* 5th ed. Philadelphia: WB Saunders, 2000. (Chapters on blood cells, spleen, and lymph nodes, good discussion of treatment of hematologic disorders in dogs and cats)

Feldman BF, Zinkl JG, Jain NC. *Schalm's Veterinary Hematology,* 5th ed. Philadelphia: Lippincott, Williams Wilkins, 2000. (This is the most complete reference text. The 5th edition is a great improvement over the older editions)

Hawkey CM, Donnett TB. *A color atlas of comparative veterinary haematology.* London: Wolfe Medical, 1989. (Good reference for nonmammalian species)

Jain NC. *Essentials of veterinary hematology.* Philadelphia: Lea & Febeger, 1993. (An abridged version of older editions of *Schalm's Veterinary Hematology.* See below)

Reagan WJ, Sanders TG, DeNicola DB. *Veterinary hematology, atlas of common domestic species.* Ames: Iowa State University Press, 1998. (Color photographs of normal and abnormal morphology of blood cells)

Wintrobe MM. *Blood, pure and eloquent.* New York: McGraw-Hill, 1980. (Wonderful historical, philosophical, documentary on the field of hematology by a father of the field)

Questions

1. A decreased total protein level in an anemic patient could indicate:

   (A) Congenital red cell enzyme deficiency
   (B) Oxidative toxins
   (C) Immune-mediated hemolysis
   (D) Aplastic anemia
   (E) Blood loss

2. Which of the following can return to the circulation after traveling in the tissues?

   (A) Neutrophils
   (B) Eosinophils
   (C) Lymphocytes
   (D) Reticulocytes
   (E) Platelets

3. One of the classic experiments in hematology involved the injection of genetically identical marrow cells into lethally irradiated mice. Survivors initially developed foci of hematopoiesis in the spleen and marrow. The most important finding from this experiment is that:

   (A) The marrow cells of the irradiated animals survived
   (B) The major source of stem cells is in the spleen
   (C) Radiation does not destroy growth factors
   (D) The spleen is an important site of hematopoiesis in adult animals
   (E) Pluripotent stem cells can differentiate to any hematopoietic cell line

4. Which of the following is present in greatest number in the marrow?

   (A) Myeloblasts
   (B) Mature neutrophils
   (C) Mature lymphocytes
   (D) Rubriblasts
   (E) Megakaryocytes

5. The red cell life span in mammals:

   (A) Averages 10–20 days in most animals
   (B) Is shortened in cases of hemolytic anemia
   (C) Is longest in the largest animals
   (D) Is determined by hematopoietic growth factors
   (E) Is about the same as that of neutrophils

6. The *lowest* circulating erythropoietin concentration would be found in an animal with:

   (A) No disease (normal animal)
   (B) Iron deficiency anemia
   (C) Chronic renal failure

   (D) Primary bone marrow failure
   (E) Congenital red cell enzyme deficiency

7. An anemic dog has a RBC count of $2 \times 10^6/\mu L$ and an observed reticulocyte count of 1.5%. Which conclusion can be drawn?

   (A) The anemia is hemolytic and regenerative
   (B) The anemia is regenerative but cause cannot be determined
   (C) The anemia is nonregenerative
   (D) No conclusion can be drawn without knowing the Hct
   (E) No conclusion can be drawn without knowing indices

8. A cat is seen in your clinic because of progressive weakness over the past 4 days. The mucous membranes are very pale and the Hct is found to be 9%. The WBC is $3,000/\mu L$ with 20 nucleated red cells per 100 white cells. The reticulocyte count is 4% aggregate and 15% punctate. Your conclusion is that the anemia:

   (A) Is regenerative because of increased aggregate and punctate reticulocytes
   (B) Is regenerative because of increased nucleated red cells
   (C) Is regenerative because of increased punctate reticulocytes
   (D) Is nonregenerative
   (E) Cannot be classified as to regenerative or nonregenerative because it is too acute

9. When blood is stored for later transfusions, the concentration of 2,3-DPG decreases over time. The impact of this on the eventual recipient of the transfusion is that:

   (A) Tissue oxygenation is increased
   (B) Binding of oxygen to hemoglobin is increased
   (C) Uptake of oxygen in the lungs is decreased
   (D) Aerobic metabolism is utilized in red cells
   (E) Increased utilization of the hexose monophosphate shunt occurs

10. Mature red cells utilize:

    (A) The Krebs-TCA cycle and heme synthesis
    (B) RNA synthesis and heme synthesis
    (C) The Embden-Meyerhof pathway and hexose monophosphate shunt
    (D) The Embden-Meyerhof pathway and Krebs-TCA cycle
    (E) The hexose monophosphate shunt and DNA synthesis

11. **Which of the following is true about hemoglobin?**

    (A) Mature red cells can produce additional heme as needed
    (B) Globin molecules have identical amino acid structures for all species
    (C) Iron is normally in the Fe^{3+} state in hemoglobin
    (D) Each molecule of hemoglobin is 1 heme unit and 2 α- and 2 β-globin chains
    (E) The region where the 2 αβ dimers come in contact is where oxygen binding takes place

12. **The oxygen dissociation curve shifts to the right to release oxygen more easily in situations of:**

    (A) Decreased pH
    (B) Decreased 2,3-DPG
    (C) Decreased temperature
    (D) Decreased carbon dioxide
    (E) Methemoglobinemia

13. **As red cells age:**

    (A) Decreased ATP causes increased rigidity of the membrane
    (B) They are removed in the marrow
    (C) The hemoglobin content decreases
    (D) Oxidative metabolism decreases
    (E) They can no longer take up oxygen in the lungs

14. **Increased serum concentrations of bilirubin might be found in all of the following conditions *except:***

    (A) Biliary obstruction
    (B) Acute hepatitis
    (C) Intravascular hemolysis
    (D) Extravascular hemolysis
    (E) Urethral obstruction

15. **The best indicator of the *variation* of red cell size is the:**

    (A) MCV
    (B) Hct
    (C) Reticulocyte count
    (D) MCHC
    (E) RDW

16. **If you knew that an animal had an MCV of 70 fL and a Hct of 30%, you could say that:**

    (A) The red cell count is $4.3 \times 10^6/\mu L$
    (B) The anemia is regenerative
    (C) The animal is probably a dog
    (D) The MCHC is 21 gm/dL
    (E) You need more information before saying any of the above

17. **A normal Hct and a high TP concentration indicate:**

    (A) Hyperglobulinemia
    (B) Anemia and dehydration
    (C) Erythroleukemia and lipemia
    (D) Dehydration alone
    (E) Either A or B

18. **All of the following are valid morphological descriptions of anemia *except:***

    (A) Macrocytic hyperchromic
    (B) Macrocytic normochromic
    (C) Macrocytic hypochromic
    (D) Microcytic hypochromic
    (E) Normocytic normochromic

19. **A previously healthy dog was hit by a car and lost a large amount of blood from a deep cut in the thigh. Twenty-four hours later, the Hct was 28% and the reticulocyte count was 0.5%. These findings are most likely indicative of:**

    (A) Acute iron deficiency
    (B) Pure red cell aplasia
    (C) Ineffective erythropoiesis
    (D) A normal marrow response
    (E) Anemia of chronic disease

20. **All of the following occur as compensatory mechanisms after acute severe blood loss *except:***

    (A) Movement of interstitial fluid to the vascular space
    (B) Splenic contraction
    (C) Tachypnea
    (D) Tachycardia
    (E) Peripheral vasodilatation

21. **When aging red cells are removed from the circulation of a normal animal, the majority of the iron is:**

    (A) Transported to the marrow
    (B) Stored in the liver
    (C) Excreted in the urine
    (D) Excreted in the bile
    (E) Stored in the spleen

22. **Total iron-binding capacity and percent saturation are sometimes used to evaluate a patient for iron deficiency. The percent saturation measures the relative percentage of iron-binding sites on _____ that are occupied.**

    (A) Ferritin
    (B) Transferrin
    (C) Hemosiderin
    (D) Haptoglobin
    (E) Lactoferrin

23. If an anemic monkey had a Hct of 20% and an MCHC of 25 gm/dL, which of the following is most likely?

(A) Iron deficiency is a likely diagnosis
(B) The Hb is 8 gm/dL
(C) The anemia is nonregenerative
(D) An artifact such as lipemia is present
(E) No conclusion can be drawn without knowing normal values

24. An *early* indicator of iron deficiency is:

(A) Reticulocytopenia
(B) Increased serum ferritin
(C) Microcytic hypochromic anemia
(D) Loss of marrow iron stores
(E) Decreased RDW

25. The best evidence of *intravascular* hemolysis is:

(A) Spherocytosis
(B) Schistocytosis
(C) Icterus
(D) Reticulocytosis
(E) Hemoglobinemia

26. A 4-year-old female terrier has had progressive weakness over the past week. On physical examination she is found to be pale and slightly icteric. The laboratory data are as follows:

Hct   24%
MCV   95 fL
MCHC   29 gm/dL
Reticulocyte count 23%

The plasma is yellow. Polychromasia, anisocytosis, and a few spherocytes are seen. What is the most likely reason for the macrocytosis?

(A) Folate or B$_{12}$ deficiency
(B) Myelodysplasia
(C) Retroviral infection
(D) Reticulocytosis
(E) Artifact

27. For the same 4-year-old female terrier described in the previous question, what test might yield the most useful information?

(A) Bone marrow aspiration
(B) Bone marrow biopsy
(C) Serum iron measurement
(D) Coombs' test
(E) Folate and cobalamin measurements

28. The best evidence for immune-mediated hemolysis is:

(A) Autoagglutination
(B) Schistocytosis
(C) Icterus
(D) Reticulocytosis
(E) Hemoglobinemia

29. Which of the following transfusions would be the safest for the recipient? (Consider both antibody sensitization and hemolytic transfusion reaction.)

(A) A-positive equine blood given to an A-negative horse
(B) B-positive feline blood given to an A-positive cat
(C) A-negative canine blood given to an A-positive dog
(D) A-positive feline blood given to a B-positive cat
(E) Rh-positive human blood given to an Rh-negative person

30. In most domestic species, hemolytic disease of the newborn animal typically occurs:

(A) In utero, even during a first pregnancy, from preformed maternal antibodies against fetal red cells
(B) When a newborn animal with autoantibodies that cross-react with maternal red cells begins to nurse
(C) At about 3–4 weeks of age when milk contains the highest titers of antibodies against the newborn's red cells
(D) In the first 1 or 2 days of life when maternal antibodies against red cells of the sire and newborn are ingested
(E) In utero when antibodies to fetal red cells have developed after multiple pregnancies

31. An advantage of red cell transfusion over the use of purified hemoglobin is that:

(A) Red cells survive longer in the circulation
(B) Typing and crossmatching are easier
(C) Red cells can be stored longer
(D) Red cells have better perfusion of poorly vascularized tissues
(E) Red cells can be given to other species (e.g., dog red cells can be given to cats)

32. An anemic dog has been given a transfusion with hemoglobin solution. The day after the transfusion, the total Hb measured from the dog's blood is 10 gm/dL. The plasma Hb is 6 gm/dL. What is the dog's Hct? (Assume a normal MCV and MCHC.)

(A) 16%
(B) 12%
(C) 10%
(D) 6%
(E) 4%

33. Which of the following occurs as a result of oxidant toxicity to red cells?

(A) Methemoglobinemia
(B) Spherocytosis
(C) Increased concentration of reduced glutathione
(D) Heme iron in the ferrous (2+) state
(E) Döhle bodies

34. **Precipitated denatured hemoglobin in red cells may be referred to as:**

(A) Döhle bodies
(B) Heinz bodies
(C) Howell-Jolly bodies
(D) Basophilic stippling
(E) Toxic granules

35. **A cat with hemobartonellosis has a red cell count of $4.5 \times 10^6/\mu L$ and an aggregate reticulocyte count of 4%. What conclusion can be drawn?**

(A) *Haemobartonella* organisms interfere with counting aggregate reticulocytes on Wright's stain
(B) *Haemobartonella* organisms interfere with counting aggregate reticulocytes on new methylene blue stain
(C) The anemia is regenerative
(D) The anemia is nonregenerative
(E) No conclusion can be drawn without knowing the Hct

36. **Equine infectious anemia is:**

(A) Caused by a retrovirus
(B) Associated with reticulocytosis and icterus
(C) Also called red water disease because of severe hemoglobinuria
(D) More common in splenectomized horses
(E) Associated with methemoglobinemia

37. **Which of the following conditions is most likely to be associated with schistocytes on a blood smear?**

(A) Splenic hemangiosarcoma
(B) Oxidative toxicity to red cells
(C) Congenital pyruvate kinase deficiency
(D) Lymphoma
(E) Polycythemia vera

38. **A dog with which of the following conditions is likely to have the largest MCV?**

(A) Aplastic anemia
(B) Polycythemia vera
(C) Anemia secondary to renal failure
(D) Iron deficiency anemia
(E) Hemolytic anemia from zinc toxicity

39. **Which of the following is most typical of nonregenerative anemia secondary to marrow failure?**

(A) Increased RDW
(B) Normocytic normochromic anemia
(C) Polychromasia
(D) Decreased erythropoietin
(E) Coexisting leukocytosis

40. **A very emaciated and dehydrated cat returned home after disappearing for 2 weeks. The rectal temperature is 98°F (normal 101–102°F), and dark bloody soft stool is present on the thermometer. The following hemogram is obtained:**

Hct	12%
WBC	500/μL
Total protein	9 gm/dL
Platelet count	20,000/μL

Which of the following diagnoses is most likely?

(A) Chronic lymphocytic leukemia
(B) Immune-mediated hemolytic anemia
(C) Bone marrow failure
(D) Intestinal parasites
(E) Myeloma

41. **Anemia of chronic disease typically is characterized by:**

(A) Decreased marrow iron stores
(B) Reticulocytosis
(C) Hematocrit <15%
(D) Reversibility if disease resolves
(E) Progression to marrow fibrosis

42. **The primary mechanism that causes anemia of chronic disease is:**

(A) Iron deficiency in the diet
(B) Impaired transfer of iron from macrophages to red cell precursors
(C) Utilization of host iron by bacteria
(D) Depletion of ferritin
(E) Inability of apoferritin to bind oxygen

43. **Animals with chronic renal failure are usually anemic. The best treatment for this type of anemia is:**

(A) Iron supplementation
(B) IL-3
(C) Erythropoietin
(D) Dialysis to remove waste products
(E) Folic acid and vitamin B$_{12}$

44. **The anemia of renal failure is:**

(A) Macrocytic normochromic
(B) A hemolytic anemia caused by changes in red cell membranes
(C) Caused by decreased production of erythropoietin by the glomerulus
(D) An indication that renal failure is chronic
(E) More severe because of low 2,3-DPG

45. **The most common cause of cobalamin deficiency in dogs is:**

(A) Decreased gastric production of intrinsic factor
(B) Intestinal bacterial overgrowth
(C) Dietary deficiency
(D) Inhibition by chemotherapeutic drugs
(E) Inherited malabsorption

46. Some chemotherapeutic drugs inhibit dihydrofolate reductase. The most important result of this is:

(A) Megaloblastic anemia
(B) Decreased synthesis of DNA
(C) Decreased homocystine production
(D) Inability to absorb tetrahydrofolate
(E) Decreased methionine production

47. The most common cause of severe red cell hypoplasia in the cat is:

(A) Feline leukemia virus
(B) Drugs or chemicals in the environment
(C) Iatrogenic
(D) Secondary to chronic bacterial infection
(E) End-stage renal disease

48. The most frequent presenting sign in dogs with ehrlichiosis is:

(A) Epistaxis
(B) Vomiting and diarrhea
(C) Cystitis secondary to neutropenia
(D) Icterus
(E) Hemarthrosis

49. Which of the following is most likely to cause aplastic anemia in the dog?

(A) Sertoli cell tumor
(B) Hepatic carcinoma
(C) Renal carcinoma
(D) Myeloma
(E) Hemangiosarcoma

50. Phenylbutazone can cause aplastic anemia in dogs. What is likely to be the first abnormality in the hemogram?

(A) Thrombocytopenia
(B) Monocytopenia
(C) Nucleated red cells
(D) Nonregenerative anemia
(E) Neutropenia

51. Retroviruses are likely to cause all of the following except:

(A) Acute leukemia
(B) Lymphoma
(C) Immunosuppression
(D) Heinz body anemia
(E) Bone marrow suppression

52. Bone marrow aspiration or biopsy would be most helpful in providing useful information in which of the following situations?

(A) Nonregenerative anemia with renal failure
(B) Acute hemolytic anemia of unknown cause
(C) Eosinophilia of unknown cause

(D) Leukocytosis with a left shift of unknown cause
(E) Pancytopenia of unknown cause

53. A patient presents with a Hct of 80% and a total protein level of 7.0 gm/dL. Cardiac and pulmonary function are normal. Which of the following would be of most value in differentiating polycythemia vera from polycythemia secondary to a renal tumor?

(A) A trial dose of intravenous fluids
(B) Bone marrow aspiration
(C) Red cell count
(D) Hemoglobin concentration
(E) Erythropoietin concentration

54. A dog has a Hct of 80%. Which of the following would help distinguish a relative polycythemia (no increase in red cell mass) from an absolute polycythemia?

(A) Elevated red cell count
(B) Elevated hemoglobin concentration
(C) Clinical signs of weakness and red mucous membranes
(D) A normal bone marrow (M/E ratio = 1)
(E) Leukocytosis

55. A cat presents with the following:

Hct   20%
WBC   1,500/μL
Differential count   10% neutrophils, 50% lymphocytes, 10% monocytes, 30% eosinophils

Considering the leukogram, which of the following is present?

(A) Eosinophilia
(B) Lymphocytosis
(C) Lymphopenia
(D) Monocytosis
(E) A and B

56. If a WBC count is 10,000/μL with 200 nucleated red cells per 100 WBCs on the differential count, what is the "corrected" WBC count/μL?

(A) 10,000
(B) 9,800
(C) 6,667
(D) 5,000
(E) 3,333

57. The absolute neutrophil count in a hemogram represents neutrophil numbers in the:

(A) Circulating pool
(B) Marginated pool
(C) Storage pool
(D) A and B
(E) A, B, and C

58. **When inflammation occurs, the number of circulating neutrophils increases. Which is the *least* likely source of this response?**

(A) Release of the marginated pool
(B) Release of the marrow storage pool
(C) Release of immature neutrophils from the marrow
(D) Recruitment of tissue neutrophils back to the circulation
(E) Recruitment of more marrow myelocytes to divide

59. **A calf is diagnosed with bovine leukocyte adhesion defect. Which of the following is most characteristic?**

(A) Chronic viral respiratory infection
(B) Recurring intestinal helminth parasites
(C) Recurring staphylococcal gingivitis
(D) Persistent neutropenia
(E) Decreased white cell production in the marrow

60. **Which of the following might be seen in response to an injection of a glucocorticoid drug in a patient with rheumatoid arthritis?**

(A) Increased chemotactic response of neutrophils
(B) Increased secretion of G-CSF
(C) Decreased movement of neutrophils from the circulation to tissues
(D) Increased margination of neutrophils
(E) Neutropenia

61. **A CBC for a cow with a febrile illness of unknown cause showed:**

Hct	32%
WBC	3,200/μL
Segs	980/μL
Bands	1,500/μL
Metas	120/μL
Lymphocytes	600/μL
Platelets	150,000/μL

Your interpretation of the leukocyte count is:

(A) Glucocorticoid stress
(B) Acute overwhelming inflammation
(C) A and B
(D) Marrow failure as the primary effect of a virus
(E) Chronic inflammation

62. **Which of the following is most useful in differentiating an epinephrine response from a corticosteroid response?**

(A) Total white blood cell count
(B) Neutrophil count
(C) Lymphocyte count
(D) Presence or absence of bands
(E) Basophil count

63. **When cells are produced in the marrow, the 2 cell lines that develop most closely together are:**

(A) Neutrophils and eosinophils
(B) Neutrophils and lymphocytes
(C) Monocytes and lymphocytes
(D) Neutrophils and red cells
(E) Neutrophils and monocytes

64. **A patient received a myelosuppressive drug that caused pancytopenia. Today, for the first time, monocytosis is present. What is the most likely interpretation?**

(A) The marrow is beginning to recover
(B) This is an adverse prognostic sign of permanent damage
(C) A secondary infection is present
(D) These monocytes probably came from the spleen
(E) Malignant changes are occurring in the marrow

65. **Eosinophils play an important role in host defense against:**

(A) Viruses
(B) Bacteria
(C) Fungi
(D) Nematodes
(E) Protozoa

66. **The following leukogram is obtained from a 2-year-old dog with a cough.**

WBC	14,000/μL
Segs	8,000
Bands	200
Lymphocytes	3,000
Eosinophils	2,800

A diagnosis that would be most compatible with these data is:

(A) Viral pneumonia
(B) Bacterial pneumonia
(C) Allergic bronchitis
(D) Neoplasia
(E) Hyperadrenocorticism with secondary infection

67. **On a smear of blood from a cat with *severe* splenomegaly, you see several cells with round nuclei and multiple purple granules. The rest of the smear appears normal. The most likely diagnosis is:**

(A) Hypersplenism
(B) Basophilic leukemia
(C) Mast cell tumor
(D) Infiltration with eosinophils and basophils
(E) Splenic abscess with toxic neutrophils

68. **When basophilia is indicated by a leukogram, you might also expect to see:**

(A) Neutrophilia
(B) Eosinophilia

(C) Monocytosis
(D) Lymphocytosis
(E) A left shift

69. **Which of the early bone marrow progenitors separates from others at the earliest stage of development (i.e., just beyond the pluripotent stem cell)?**

(A) Red cells
(B) Neutrophils
(C) Lymphocytes
(D) Monocytes
(E) Megakaryocytes

70. **The immunosuppressive effects of retroviruses such as HIV and FIV are largely mediated by loss of:**

(A) Function of all lymphocytes despite normal numbers
(B) B cells
(C) Natural killer cells
(D) CD8$^+$ T cells
(E) CD4$^+$ T cells

71. **A 12-year-old dog has the following findings on a hemogram:**

Hct	38%
WBC	75,000/μL
Neutrophils	13,000
Lymphocytes	60,000
Monocytes	1,400
Eosinophils	600
Platelets	200,000/μL

Red and white cell morphology is normal. The most likely diagnosis is:

(A) Acute lymphoblastic leukemia
(B) Chronic lymphocytic leukemia
(C) Epinephrine response
(D) Leukemoid response
(E) Viral lymphocytosis

72. **In a health survey of a herd of dairy cattle, several are found to have significant lymphocytosis. The lymphocytes appear normal, and the rest of the CBC is normal. A possible cause that should be investigated is:**

(A) Lymphocytic leukemia
(B) Bovine leukemia virus infection
(C) Epinephrine effect
(D) Chronic bacterial infection
(E) Addison's disease (Hypoedrenocortism)

73. **Which of the following terms best defines lymphadenopathy?**

(A) Lymphoma
(B) Nonspecific lymph node enlargement
(C) Necrotizing lymphadenitis

(D) Reactive hyperplasia of lymph nodes
(E) Granulomatous lymphadenitis

74. **The histopathology report on the lymph node biopsy specimen you submitted reads as follows: "This lymph node shows essentially normal architecture with a prominent follicular pattern and large cortical germinal centers. Many lymphocytes and plasma cells are scattered throughout the cortex and medulla." The diagnosis is:**

(A) Reactive hyperplasia
(B) Suppurative lymphadenitis
(C) Lymphoma
(D) Lymphadenopathy
(E) Tuberculosis (granulomatous lymphadenitis)

75. **Which of the following syndromes most commonly occurs with thymoma?**

(A) T-cell suppression
(B) Hypoglycemia
(C) Immune-mediated hemolytic anemia
(D) Myasthenia gravis
(E) DiGeorge syndrome

76. **Which of the following statements regarding the thymus is correct?**

(A) It begins to regress in dogs at 5 years of age
(B) Lymphoma in this organ is called thymoma
(C) Combined immunodeficiency disease with atrophy of the thymus is common in cattle
(D) Nude mice are born without a thymus gland
(E) Thymic (Hassle's) corpuscles are composed of large histiocytic cells

77. **After splenectomy a patient is more susceptible to:**

(A) Hemangiosarcoma
(B) Eosinophilia
(C) Red cell parasites
(D) Spherocytosis
(E) Pancytopenia

78. **Which of the following is most likely to be associated with splenic hemangiosarcoma in a dog?**

(A) Incidental finding on physical exam
(B) Increased hematocrit from splenic contraction
(C) Intraabdominal hemorrhage
(D) Pancytopenia from hypersplenism
(E) Diffuse splenomegaly

79. **Which of the following substances secreted by platelet granules causes vasoconstriction?**

(A) Nitrous oxide
(B) ADP
(C) Prostacyclin
(D) von Willebrand factor
(E) Thromboxane

80. **Matrix metalloproteinase inhibitors are being tested as possible anticancer agents. They function primarily by preventing tumor cells from:**

(A) Adhering to blood vessels
(B) Producing proteins
(C) Entering blood vessels
(D) Invading tissues
(E) Multiplying at metastatic sites

81. **Following vessel injury and reflex vasoconstriction, the *initial* event in hemostatic plug formation is:**

(A) Platelet adhesion to exposed collagen
(B) Activation of clotting factors
(C) Activation of platelet factors
(D) Activation of fibrinolysis
(E) Platelet aggregation

82. **Which of the following is true regarding platelet transfusion in patients with von Willebrand disease (vWD)?**

(A) Platelet transfusion is helpful in treating bleeding because it raises the platelet count to a safe range
(B) Platelet transfusion is not helpful in treating bleeding because an autoantibody destroys transfused platelets immediately
(C) Platelet transfusion would be helpful in type 1 vWD but not in type 2 or 3
(D) A dog affected with vWD might be an effective platelet donor to another patient
(E) A dog that is a normal carrier of vWD, but not an affected dog might be an effective platelet donor

83. **The complex made up of factors Xa and Va plus phospholipid and calcium serves primarily to:**

(A) Activate vitamin K–dependent factors
(B) Convert prothrombin to thrombin
(C) Convert fibrinogen to fibrin
(D) Convert plasminogen to plasmin
(E) Activate antithrombin, protein C, and protein S

84. **Fibrin formation is initiated:**

(A) By the action of tissue plasminogen activator
(B) By the release of thromboxane A_2 by activated platelets
(C) When tissue factor is exposed to factor VII
(D) Following factor XII activation by the complex of factor XIa, prekallikrein, and high-molecular-weight kininogen

(E) By the action of the prothrombinase complex on prothrombin

85. **The protein C–protein S and heparin–antithrombin III systems function as natural anticoagulants because they inhibit the formation or activity of:**

(A) Thrombin
(B) Tissue factor
(C) Fibrin-degradation products
(D) Thromboxane A_2
(E) Plasminogen

86. **The mediator of fibrinolysis is:**

(A) Thrombin
(B) Plasmin
(C) Fibrin-degradation product fragments
(D) Antithrombin III
(E) Activated protein C

87. **You are attempting to draw a blood sample for a CBC on a Vietnamese pot-bellied pig that does not appreciate your efforts. After multiple sticks, you finally get 1 mL of blood in an EDTA tube. When you get to the laboratory, you notice that a large clot has formed in the tube. What is your response?**

(A) You used the wrong type of tube; draw another sample in citrate
(B) Submit the sample as the effects of the clot on the results are minimal
(C) Tissue factor probably contaminated your sample; try again to get a "clean" stick
(D) You will not be able to get a sample on an excited pig because epinephrine will make the blood clot quickly
(E) Blood should not clot in EDTA, so the pig must have thrombotic tendencies

88. **Why might the ACT be prolonged in an animal with severe ITP (platelet count 1,000/μL)?**

(A) Autoantibodies inactivate fibrin
(B) Platelet aggregation is needed to start clotting
(C) Platelets adhere to clay to start clotting
(D) Platelets are needed to provide calcium
(E) Platelets are needed to provide phospholipid

89. **A 5-year-old Holstein cow has petechiae on the gums and ventral part of the abdomen. These findings are suggestive of a defect in which component of the hemostatic mechanism?**

(A) Extrinsic pathway factors
(B) Plasminogen
(C) Antithrombin III
(D) Platelets
(E) Fibrinogen

90. A Good Samaritan brings you an approximately 5-month-old male beagle that appeared on a front step. It looks well nourished but is weak and has a slightly distended abdomen. When you tap it with a needle, a bloody fluid is found. You look at a blood smear and see adequate platelets. The bleeding time and ACT are normal. At this point, you suspect:

(A) Warfarin toxicity
(B) A hereditary platelet aggregation defect
(C) von Willebrand disease
(D) Hemophilia B
(E) No coagulopathy; trauma is likely

91. All of the following are associated with thrombocytopenia *except:*

(A) Acute leukemia
(B) Aplastic anemia
(C) ITP
(D) von Willebrand disease
(E) DIC

92. Which of the following best describes findings in ITP?

(A) Platelet count is usually 60–70,000/μL when the animal starts to bleed
(B) When bleeding starts, swollen joints are a common presenting sign
(C) Megakaryocytes are usually decreased in the marrow
(D) A minimal decrease in platelet number but major abnormality of platelet function is present
(E) Platelets on blood smear are often larger than normal

93. A 4-month-old male Scottish terrier has excessive bleeding from teething. The clotting test results are as follows:

	Patient	Control
Platelet count	140,000/μL	(200,000–400,000/μL)
PT	8 sec	9 sec
APTT	18 sec	16 sec
Fibrinogen concentration	250 mg/dL	200–400 mg/dL
FDP concentration	Negative	Negative

Which of the following still remains a possible cause of the bleeding?

(A) ITP
(B) von Willebrand disease
(C) Hemophilia A
(D) Factor X deficiency
(E) DIC

94. A horse treated with NSAIDs might have which of the following types of bleeding?

(A) Gastrointestinal bleeding
(B) Blood in joints
(C) Blood in the thoracic cavity
(D) Subcutaneous hematomas
(E) Subdural hematoma of the brain

95. A 4-month-old, otherwise healthy male dog had blood in the thoracic cavity. The clotting tests showed the following:

Platelet count	350,000/μL
PT	>40 sec
APTT	>40 sec
Fibrinogen	<25 mg/dL
FDPs	Negative

The most likely diagnosis is a deficiency of:

(A) Factor VII
(B) Factor VIII
(C) Fibrinogen
(D) Factors II, VII, IX, and X
(E) von Willebrand factor

96. Hemophilia A is diagnosed in an animal with a bleeding tendency that developed shortly after birth. Both the sire and dam were clinically normal. If they were bred again in the future, what would be the expected result?

(A) All males affected clinically, all females normal
(B) All males affected, all females healthy carriers
(C) Half of the males affected, all females healthy carriers
(D) All males healthy carriers, all females normal
(E) Half of the males affected, half of the females healthy carriers

97. The following hemogram is obtained for a dog with severe weakness, fever, and bloody diarrhea:

Hct	20%
Platelet count	80,000/μL
ACT	Greatly prolonged

Although a specific diagnosis has not been made, the most likely explanation for the *bleeding* is:

(A) Blood-sucking intestinal parasites
(B) ITP
(C) DIC
(D) von Willebrand disease
(E) Bone marrow failure

98. You are presented with a 3-year-old male, mixed-breed dog that is allowed to run unsupervised. On physical examination, he is found to be moderately lethargic and reluctant to move. He has fluctuant swellings on his thorax and abdomen. The coagulation profile is as follows:

	Patient	Control
PT	45 sec	6 sec
APPT	55 sec	15 sec
Fibrinogen	330 mg/dL	170 mg/dL
FDP	<10 μg/dL	—
Platelets	192,000μg/dL	—

The most probable diagnosis is:

(A) Warfarin poisoning
(B) ITP
(C) Aspirin toxicity
(D) von Willebrand disease
(E) Inherited factor VII deficiency

99. **Chronic glomerulonephritis is associated with a loss of albumin and antithrombin in the urine. A consequence could be:**

(A) Mucosal bleeding
(B) Thrombosis
(C) Loss of fibrinogen
(D) Prolonged ACT
(E) Bleeding into body cavities

100. **An important difference between arterial and venous thrombi is that venous thrombi:**

(A) Contain fewer red cells
(B) Are more likely to cause pulmonary embolism
(C) Are more likely to cause cerebral embolism
(D) Are more common in cats with cardiomyopathy
(E) Are initiated by abnormal endothelium

101. **Which of the following statements regarding leukemogenesis is true?**

(A) Aggressive leukemias usually result from simultaneous transformation of many cells in the marrow
(B) Oncogenes are foreign genes introduced into cells by viruses
(C) Activated oncogenes are often growth factors or growth factor receptors
(D) Cellular oncogenes can be activated by the *p53* gene
(E) Most changes in oncogenes are inherited

102. **To cause malignant transformation, viruses must integrate into the host DNA. The component of retroviruses that allows them to integrate is:**

(A) The ability to pick up cellular proto-oncogenes
(B) Double-stranded DNA
(C) The enzyme reverse transcriptase
(D) Growth factor receptors on the surface
(E) The ability to be transmitted in the germ line from mother to offspring

103. **A dog with lymphoma is most likely to have:**

(A) A mediastinal mass
(B) Generalized lymphadenopathy
(C) Blasts replacing the marrow
(D) A white blood count with >10,000 lymphoblasts
(E) Skin nodules

104. **As a general statement, lymphoma:**

(A) Is a polyclonal proliferation of undifferentiated lymphoblasts

(B) Is derived from T-cell areas of multiple lymph nodes
(C) Is monoclonal but can arise from any type of lymphoid progenitor
(D) Always affects the same type of lymphoid progenitor within a given species
(E) Is a B-cell disease, usually associated with monoclonal gammopathy

105. **All of the following are characteristic of any acute leukemia *except:***

(A) Malignant cells are monoclonal
(B) Malignant cells fill the marrow
(C) Malignant cells function normally
(D) Neutropenia, thrombocytopenia, and anemia occur
(E) Circulating malignant cells vary from none to very high numbers

106. **A patient with erythroleukemia is likely to have:**

(A) Anemia
(B) Polycythemia
(C) Reticulocytosis
(D) A fibrotic bone marrow
(E) A leukemoid reaction

107. **Myelodysplasia is associated primarily with:**

(A) Peripheral cytopenias and a cellular marrow
(B) Myelofibrosis
(C) A marrow filled with blasts
(D) Microcytosis and anisocytosis
(E) A leukemoid reaction

108. **Which of the following is most likely to be confused with a "leukemoid" reaction to severe inflammation?**

(A) Acute myelogenous leukemia
(B) Acute myelomonocyte leukemia
(C) Acute promyelocytic leukemia
(D) Chronic myelogenous leukemia
(E) Myelodysplasia

109. **The most likely cause of a polyclonal gammopathy is:**

(A) Myeloma
(B) Chronic infection
(C) Hyperviscosity syndrome
(D) Dehydration
(E) Either A or C

110. **Which of the following problems is most likely to occur in dogs with myeloma?**

(A) Proliferative bone lesions
(B) Prolonged ACT
(C) Decreased serum calcium concentration
(D) Polyclonal gammopathy
(E) Marrow filled with immature plasma cells

111. **A common life-threatening complication of disseminated mast cell tumor is:**

(A) Hyperviscosity
(B) Renal shutdown
(C) Seizures
(D) Pulmonary metastases
(E) Duodenal ulcers

112. **Transmissible venereal tumors in dogs most likely arise from transplanted malignant:**

(A) Histiocytes
(B) B cells
(C) T cells
(D) Fibroblasts
(E) Squamous epithelial cells

Answers

1. **The answer is E.**
When blood is lost, serum proteins are lost in equal proportion to red cells. In anemia of other causes, red cell numbers are decreased, but serum protein levels remain normal.

2. **The answer is C.**
Lymphocytes travel out of the blood and into lymphoid organs, eventually returning to the circulation via lymphatic vessels and the thoracic duct. Neutrophils and eosinophils travel to the tissues and do not return. Platelets and reticulocytes do not leave.

3. **The answer is E.**
The colonies were observed to produce progeny of all cell lines even though they started from 1 cell. The marrow cells would survive since they are genetically identical. The source of the stem cells was the donor mouse. It is true that radiation does not destroy growth factors but that was not the focus of the experiment. The spleen functioned in hematopoiesis only temporarily. Eventually the marrow takes over.

4. **The answer is B.**
Normally only a few blasts are present, with numbers progressively increasing as they mature. Lymphocytes mature primarily outside the marrow, and only a few megakaryocytes are present. Many mature neutrophils are stored in the marrow.

5. **The answer is B.**
Hemolysis is the premature destruction of red cells. Their life span normally is 90–140 days, whereas neutrophils survive only a few hours. Smaller animals have a shorter red cell life span than larger animals. Growth factors increase the number of progenitors and may speed maturation but do not affect the life span of cells.

6. **The answer is C.**
Erythropoietin is produced in the kidney and is decreased in renal failure. A steady state of erythropoietin secretion is present in normal animals to replace old cells. It is increased in anemia of any other cause.

7. **The answer is C.**
The absolute reticulocyte count (RBC $\times 10^6 \times$ reticulocyte %) is 30,000/μL. Since this is <60,000/μL, the anemia is nonregenerative.

8. **The answer is D.**
Aggregate reticulocytes are most important in determining regeneration. The corrected reticulocyte count [9/37 (normal) $\times$ 4] is just under 1% so this is nonregenerative. The punctate reticulocyte count can be corrected the

same way, but normal cats may have up to 10%. Nucleated red cells are not a sign of regeneration.

9. **The answer is B.**
A function of 2,3-DPG is to allow release of oxygen in the tissues. When it is decreased, oxygen is taken up in the lungs but not released. Tissue oxygenation is decreased. Red cells cannot utilize aerobic metabolism, and the hexose monophosphate shunt is not involved.

10. **The answer is C.**
This is the only method of energy (ATP) production. Mature red cells cannot synthesize DNA or RNA or utilize the Krebs cycle.

11. **The answer is E.**
Mature red cells cannot produce additional heme or hemoglobin. Slight species-specific differences in amino acids in globin molecules exist, whereas heme is the same. Iron is normally in the 2+ state, and each molecule of hemoglobin contains 4 heme units.

12. **The answer is A.**
See the oxygen dissociation curve in Chapter 6. The pH in the peripheral tissues is lower than in the lungs, facilitating oxygen release in the tissues. All of the other options favor decreased oxygenation of tissues.

13. **The answer is A.**
ATP functions partially to maintain flexibility in the membrane so red cells can move through small capillaries and the spleen. When ATP decreases, red cells are removed primarily in the spleen, not the marrow. Oxygen uptake and hemoglobin content are not affected, and oxidative metabolism does not occur in mature red cells.

14. **The answer is E.**
Minimal excretion of bilirubin in the normal animal occurs via the urine. All of the other options can cause icterus.

15. **The answer is E.**
The RDW shows the variation of red cell size around the mean (MCV). The other options are not involved.

16. **The answer is A.**
The MCV is the Hct/RBC count, or RBC = Hct/MCV = 4.3 $\times 10^6$/μL. We do not know if the anemia is regenerative without a reticulocyte count. The MCHC cannot be calculated without the hemoglobin value (which would be about one-third of the Hct).

17. **The answer is E.**
Both the Hct and TSP are relative measurements per vol-

ume of blood. A high TSP could indicate hyperproteinemia (including hyperglobulinemia), and dehydration could raise the Hct of an anemic animal to normal. Erythroleukemia causes a low Hct, and dehydration alone causes an increased Hct.

18. The answer is A.
Red cells cannot be hyperchromic.

19. The answer is D.
Reticulocytosis occurs 3–4 days after acute blood loss. The Hct drops slowly over 12–24 hours as fluid shifts from the interstitium to the circulation.

20. The answer is E.
Peripheral *vasoconstriction* occurs to preserve blood pressure.

21. The answer is A.
The majority of the iron goes to the marrow to be recycled into new red cells. Minimal iron is lost, and only excesses are stored in the liver or occasionally the spleen.

22. The answer is B.
Transferrin is the main binding protein for iron transport. Ferritin and hemosiderin are storage forms of iron. Haptoglobin binds free hemoglobin, and lactoferrin is of minor importance in iron metabolism.

23. The answer is A.
The MCHC, normally 30–35 gm/dL, is similar for humans, other primates, and all domestic mammals. Thus, an MCHC of 25 gm/dL probably is hypochromic. Iron deficiency is the most likely cause. MCHC = Hb/Hct, so the Hb is 5 gm/dL. We do not know if the anemia is regenerative. Lipemia would cause an artifactually increased MCHC.

24. The answer is D.
Iron stores are depleted before anything changes in the blood. Reticulocytosis also occurs if blood loss is ongoing.

25. The answer is E.
Intravascular hemolysis is characterized by hemoglobinemia and hemoglobinuria. All of the other options could be seen with extravascular hemolysis as well.

26. The answer is D.
The most common cause of macrocytosis in an anemic dog is reticulocytosis. In this dog, the reticulocyte count is high, and evidence of hemolysis (icteric plasma and spherocytes) is present.

27. The answer is D.
The presence of spherocytes in the blood of an animal with a hemolytic anemia strongly suggests a diagnosis of immune-mediated hemolytic anemia. The anemia is regenerative so we know the marrow is working. There

is no evidence of iron deficiency, and folate or cobalamin deficiency is a nonregenerative anemia.

28. The answer is A.
Autoagglutination that does not clear when saline is added is diagnostic of an immune-mediated cause if the clinical signs are compatible. Schistocytosis is indicative of microangiopathic anemia. Icterus can occur with hemolysis or liver disease of any cause. Reticulocytosis occurs with any regenerative anemia, and hemoglobinemia with any cause of intravascular hemolysis.

29. The answer is C.
A-negative blood does not introduce that antigen so it will not be a problem. Giving any (positive) antigen to a recipient lacking it will at least cause antibodies to form if they are not already there. Cats have preformed antibodies so hemolysis will occur even on the first transfusion unless the blood is of the same type.

30. The answer is D.
In animals maternal antibody against newborn red cells does not cross the placenta, but is absorbed in the first 24 hours after birth. Hemolysis then occurs within the next 1 or 2 days.

31. The answer is A.
Compatible red cells have a normal life span. Hemoglobin has a half-life of 36–48 hours. Hemoglobin does not have to be typed and can be given to other species because red cell antigens are absent. Because of hemoglobin's smaller molecular size, perfusion of ischemic tissues is better and hemoglobin can be stored longer.

32. The answer is B.
The total Hb equals the Hb in red cells plus the Hb in plasma (from transfusion). The dog's own Hb is $10 - 6$, or 4 gm/dL. Normally, Hct = Hb $\times$ 3, so the Hct is approximately 12%.

33. The answer is A.
Methemoglobin has Fe^{3+} from oxidant damage, which depletes reduced glutathione. Spherocytes and Döhle bodies are not relevant.

34. The answer is B.
This is the definition of Heinz bodies. Döhle's bodies are toxic granular inclusions in neutrophils. Howell-Jolly bodies are retained nuclear material, and basophilic stippling is ribosomal RNA in red cells.

35. The answer is C.
The absolute reticulocyte count (RBC $\times$ %reticulocytes) is 180,000/μL. If it is >60,000/μL, the anemia is regenerative. *Haemobartonella* organisms interfere with counting punctate reticulocytes on smears stained with new methylene blue.

36. The answer is A.

Equine infectious anemia does not cause oxidant damage (methemoglobinemia) or intravascular hemolysis (hemoglobinuria). Horses do not show reticulocytosis with anemia of any cause. Red water disease is a clostridial disease of cattle.

37. The answer is A.

Hemangiosarcoma fragments red cells because of abnormal vasculature and DIC. None of the other options is likely to do that.

38. The answer is E.

Hemolysis of any cause is associated with reticulocytosis (increased MCV). Aplastic anemia and renal failure cause normocytic anemia. Iron deficiency is microcytic, and polycythemia vera is associated with normal-sized mature red cells.

39. The answer is B.

Because the anemia is normocytic normochromic, the RDW is normal and polychromasia is not seen. Erythropoietin is increased, and leukopenia may be present.

40. The answer is C.

Pancytopenia is present, implying a primary bone marrow problem. The fever is probably caused by bacterial sepsis from neutropenia. The high protein level is probably from dehydration.

41. The answer is D.

The anemia is typically mild (Hct >20%) and nonregenerative with increased iron stores. It is reversible if the underlying disease improves.

42. The answer is B.

Iron is present but is not utilized. It is bound to apoferritin. Serum ferritin may be increased.

43. The answer is C.

The reason for the anemia is decreased erythropoietin, which persists even if dialysis is used. Replacement of exogenous erythropoietin restores the Hct to normal.

44. The answer is D.

If erythropoietin decreases acutely, red cells currently present would survive normally and it would take time for a significant drop in the Hct to occur. Erythropoietin is produced in peritubular cells, and the anemia is typically normocytic, normochromic, and nonregenerative. The concentration of 2,3-DPG is increased in a partially compensatory manner.

45. The answer is B.

Excessive intestinal bacteria produce folate but deplete cobalamin. Dogs do not have gastric intrinsic factor. Dietary deficiency and inherited malabsorption are rare. Some chemotherapeutic drugs inhibit folate, not cobalamin.

46. The answer is B.

Dihydrofolate reductase is an enzyme needed to produce tetrahydrofolate, which is needed to produce thymidylate as part of DNA synthesis. Megaloblastic anemia rarely occurs.

47. The answer is A.

Feline leukemia virus is a much more common cause than any of the others. Chronic infection usually causes mild anemia. Renal failure is probably the second most common cause.

48. The answer is A.

Thrombocytopenia is the most common cytopenia seen and results in mucosal bleeding, often from the nose. Neutropenia can occur but is less common.

49. The answer is A.

Sertoli cell tumors typically secrete estrogen, which causes marrow damage. None of the other options cause aplasia.

50. The answer is E.

Because neutrophils have the shortest life span, they will be the first to decrease in number if production stops.

51. The answer is D.

Heinz bodies form from oxidant damage of hemoglobin. All the other options are caused by retroviruses.

52. The answer is E.

Pancytopenia often implies that the marrow is the source of the problem. Hemolysis, eosinophilia, and leukocytosis probably would show only increased erythroid eosinophil and granulocyte precursors in the marrow, without indicating a cause.

53. The answer is E.

Polycythemia vera has a normal to low erythropoietin concentration. Renal tumors can cause polycythemia by secreting excessive erythropoietin. The red cell count is high, and erythroid hyperplasia occurs in the marrow with both conditions. The normal protein level makes dehydration unlikely.

54. The answer is D.

Relative polycythemia, as might occur in dehydration, is not associated with an increase in red cell production, so erythroid hyperplasia is not seen. The increased red cell count and hemoglobin concentration, in addition to the clinical signs noted, would occur with either condition. Leukocytosis is independent.

55. The answer is C.

Use the percentages to calculate the absolute counts of all white blood cell type. The absolute counts which are low for all WBCs are used to describe abnormalities.

56. The answer is E.
The white blood count must be "corrected" for nucleated red cells counted as white cells. When 100 white blood cells were counted, 200 nucleated red cells were counted as well. So 100/(100 + 200) is the true number of nucleated cells that are truly white cells. The white blood count is actually

$$\frac{100}{100 + 200} \times 10,000 = 3{,}333/\mu L.$$

56. The answer is B.
H_2O_2, myeloperoxidase, and HOCl are active and irritating to normal tissues. Superoxide dismutase suppresses the irritating effects of superoxide.

57. The answer is A.
Only the circulating pool is sampled.

58. The answer is D.
Neutrophils never re-enter the circulation under any circumstances.

59. The answer is C.
Neutrophilia and recurring bacterial infections occur because neutrophils do not adhere to the endothelium and get to the tissues. Neutrophils are not the major defense against viruses or helminths.

60. The answer is C.
Glucocorticoids cause neutrophilia partially because of decreased chemotaxis. No change in margination or production of neutrophils occurs.

61. The answer is C.
A left shift indicates inflammation, and lymphopenia and eosinopenia indicate glucocorticoid effect. Cattle with inflammation are more likely to show neutropenia and a severe left shift. If it were seen in a dog or cat, it would indicate overwhelming infection. Marrow failure is less likely with near-normal Hct and platelet values.

62. The answer is C.
Lymphocyte count is normal or increased with an epinephrine response and decreased with a corticosteroid response.

63. The answer is E.
GM-CSF stimulates both neutrophils and monocytes.

64. The answer is A.
Monocytes mature more quickly than neutrophils, so they appear first. The spleen does not contribute effectively to replacing cells not made in the marrow.

65. The answer is D.
Eosinophils play a major role in defense against nematodes, other parasites, and allergies.

66. The answer is C.
Eosinophilia is the primary abnormality with a mild left shift of neutrophils. Allergies or parasites most likely would be the causes.

67. The answer is C.
A major morphological difference between basophils and mast cells is that mast cells have a round nucleus and basophils a lobular nucleus. See also Chapter 57.

68. The answer is B.
The stimuli for basophils tend to be the same as for eosinophils.

69. The answer is C.
Lymphocytes develop separately from other cells beyond the stem cell level.

70. The answer is E.
The numbers of helper T cells (CD4$^+$) gradually drop, resulting in immunosuppression. Changes in other lymphocyte subtypes are less likely to occur.

71. The answer is B.
This degree of lymphocytosis is not likely to be reactive and is characteristic of chronic lymphocytic leukemia.

72. The answer is B.
Persistent lymphocytosis is a common manifestation in otherwise healthy cattle in a herd with endemic bovine leukemia virus infection. Both lymphocytic leukemia and Addison's disease are rare and sporadic. Epinephrine would induce neutrophilia as well. Bacterial infection does not typically cause lymphocytosis.

73. The answer is B.
This is the definition of lymphadenopathy. The others could cause lymphadenopathy, however.

74. The answer is A.
This description is of a hyperplastic node responding to an antigen. Neutrophils would be present in the case of suppurative lymphadenitis; a homogeneous population of lymphocytes with loss of architecture, in the case of lymphoma; and macrophages, in the case of tuberculosis.

75. The answer is D.
Antibodies against acetylcholine receptors are part of a common paraneoplastic syndrome. Since thymomas occur in older animals in which the thymus has normally involuted, T-cell function is not affected.

76. The answer is D.
Athymic nude mice (identifiable because they do not have hair) are useful in cancer research.

77. The answer is C.
The spleen normally removes red cell parasites.

78. The answer is C.
The tumor is commonly a large friable irregular mass on the spleen. It often reptures spontaneously or after minor trauma, resulting in intraabdominal hemorrhage

79. The answer is E.
Nitrous oxide and prostacyclin cause vasodilation. ADP and von Willebrand factor affect platelets.

80. The answer is D.
Matrix metalloproteinases break down collagen and allow tumor cells to invade. In addition, they have an angiogenic effect.

81. The answer is A.
All of the other options follow platelet adhesion.

82. The answer is D.
Platelets are normal in patients with vWD, but the lack of endothelial vWF interferes with their ability to adhere to areas of endothelial damage. The platelet count is normal, and abnormal antibodies are not involved. Transfusion with vWF is needed for treatment.

83. The answer is B.
This is the common pathway that, when activated, activates prothrombin.

84. The answer is C.
Damaged endothelium releases tissue factor, which binds to factor VII and activates both intrinsic and extrinsic pathways. This works much faster than activation of factor XII.

85. The answer is A.
Thrombin is inhibited before it acts to induce the conversion of fibrinogen to fibrin.

86. The answer is B.
Plasmin is the active mediator. Antithrombin III, protein C, and fibrin-degradation products prevent thrombin formation but do not break down clots.

87. The answer is C.
Trauma to the vessel causes tissue factor to mix with the blood and cause coagulation before EDTA can prevent it. The sample will have to be redrawn to prevent artifacts.

88. The answer is E.
For the ACT, formation of a clot requires phospholipid from platelets. Otherwise clotting is initiated from contact with the material in the tube.

89. The answer is D.
Any time petechiae or ecchymoses are present, an abnormality of platelets is the most likely cause. This type of bleeding occurs rarely with vascular abnormalities, but not with clotting factor abnormalities.

90. The answer is E.
Normal bleeding time rules out platelet function problems, such as vWD, and the normal ACT rules out warfarin toxicity and hemophilia.

91. The answer is D.
The platelet count is normal in von Willebrand disease and low in the others listed.

92. The answer is E.
Large platelets are usually young platelets recently released from the increased number of megakaryocytes in the marrow, and they function well. For that reason, ITP usually is not associated with bleeding until the count is very low, usually <20,000/μL. Bleeding is usually mucosal.

93. The answer is B.
The platelet count is too high to cause bleeding if platelet function is normal. A bleeding time would be necessary to rule out von Willebrand disease. The normal PT and A-PTT make factor deficiencies unlikely. A slight increase in FDPs might occur with ongoing bleeding at deeper sites.

94. The answer is A.
NSAIDs interfere with platelet function and might also cause gastric erosions.

95. The answer is C.
Fibrinogen is at the end of the common pathway, and if missing, both the PT and APTT will be prolonged. Hypofibrinogenemia is a rare inherited disease. In all of the other possibilities, fibrinogen concentration would be normal or increased.

96. The answer is E.
One affected X chromosome probably came from the dam. If she is bred to a normal male, half of the offspring would get the abnormal X chromosome. Of those, the females would be healthy carriers since they have 1 normal X chromosome, and the males would be affected.

97. The answer is C.
The platelet count is not low enough to cause bleeding by itself. The prolonged ACT indicates factor abnormalities as well. This combination in a very sick dog is probably DIC.

98. The answer is A.
Prolongation of both the PT and the APTT imply either multiple factor problems (as in vitamin K deficiency from warfarin) or common-pathway factor deficiency.

99. The answer is B.
Antithrombin is an important anticoagulant.

100. The answer is B.
Venous thrombi start in normal vessels with abnormal circulation. They contain many red cells and are easily fragmented, with emboli traveling to the right side of the heart and then to the lungs where they lodge. Cats with cardiomyopathy are more likely to have systemic thromboemboli.

101. The answer is C.
Oncogenes arise from acquired changes in normal cellular proto-oncogenes that are caused by translocations, or mutations. Activated oncogenes may promote unregulated cell growth and division, usually of 1 cell from which the tumor arises. The *p53* gene is a suppressor gene that inhibits cell growth or induces cell death.

102. The answer is C.
The characteristic of the retroviruses that are RNA viruses is the ability of reverse transcriptase to transcribe a DNA proviral copy that can insert into the host genome. The major retroviruses of humans and domestic animals are transmitted horizontally rather than vertically. The ability to pick up cellular proto-oncogenes occurs only after integration.

103. The answer is B.
The majority of dogs with lymphoma initially present with enlarged lymph nodes. Other sites are involved less often.

104. The answer is C.
Lymphoma more often affects either B or T cells depending on the species, but both types of lymphoma can be seen in any given species.

105. The answer is C.
In acute leukemia, blasts proliferate and fill the marrow but do not mature or function normally. Pancytopenia with variable numbers of circulating blasts is seen.

106. The answer is A.
Even though this is a malignancy of erythroid cells, blasts fill the marrow but do not mature to functional red cells.

107. The answer is A.
The marrow has precursors of all cell lines, but their maturation is abnormal and many die before reaching the circulation. Because of this, cytopenias occur. Later, myelodysplasia may progress to acute leukemia.

108. The answer is D.
Both CML and severe inflammation (leukemoid reaction) cause severe neutrophilia with a significant left shift. In chronic myelogenous leukemia, this may occur with minimal signs of illness, whereas patients with a leukemoid response usually have a very severe infection.

109. The answer is B.
Whatever causes an infection often has several antigens and stimulates many clones of plasma cells. Both myeloma and hyperviscosity cause a monoclonal gammopathy.

110. The answer is E.
Plasma cells secrete a monoclonal globulin and infiltrate the marrow. Bone lesions are lytic, and serum calcium levels sometimes are increased. Platelet aggregation may be abnormal, but not the ACT.

111. The answer is E.
Ulcers are caused by increased secretion of hydrochloric acid in the stomach in response to histamine in mast cell granules. Mast cell tumors rarely affect the lungs, brain, or kidneys.

112. The answer is A.
The tumor cells are bizarre histiocytes with decreased chromosomes.

Index